Beat Cancer with Anti-Cancer Juicing Recipes: 150+ Mouthwatering Recipes for Detox and Nourishment

Unique Kade

Table of Contents

Chapter 1

Introduction:

Imagine hearing the words **"You have cancer."** Your life, as you know it, will never be the same again. The journey that follows is full of **fear, uncertainty, and heartbreak.** It's a road that is often lonely, and it's easy to feel like you have lost control over your health and your life.

But what if I told you that there is a way to take control back? A way to arm yourself with the tools you need to fight back against cancer and increase your chances of beating it? That's where juicing comes in.

Juicing can be a game-changer in the fight against cancer. It's not just a fad or a trend – it's backed by science. Certain fruits and vegetables contain compounds that have been shown to have anti-cancer properties. By incorporating these foods into your diet in the form of delicious and nutritious juices, you can give your body the nutrients it needs to fight back against cancer and increase your chances of success.

In this book, we'll explore the powerful science behind juicing and its role in beating cancer. We'll provide you with **over 150 recipes** that are designed to support healing and wellness and are packed with cancer-fighting nutrients to give you the best possible chance of success. From the immune-boosting Citrus Zinger to the antioxidant-rich Berry Boost, each recipe is carefully crafted to provide your body with the vitamins, minerals, and phytochemicals that it needs to heal and thrive.

But this book is about more than just juicing – it's about hope. It's about taking an active role and controlling your health and well-being and finding strength in the face of adversity. and giving yourself the best possible **chance to beat cancer.**

Each sip is a symbol of your strength and determination, a small but powerful step on the road to recovery. **So let's raise a glass to life, to health, and to the power of juicing to beat cancer together, one sip at a time.** Together, we can give cancer a fight it will never forget.

Are you ready to take **control of your health** and fight back against cancer? If your answer is yes, **let's dive in!**

- **Benefits Of Juicing As A Complementary Therapy For Cancer Treatment.**

Juicing has gained popularity as a complementary therapy for cancer treatment. Many cancer patients incorporate fresh juices into their diet to help manage symptoms and improve overall health. While juicing should not be seen as a replacement for conventional cancer treatments, it can offer a range of benefits supporting the body during cancer treatment.

One of the primary benefits of juicing is that it can help increase the intake of essential nutrients.

Cancer treatment can weaken the immune system and cause side effects such as nausea and difficulty swallowing, making it challenging for patients to eat a balanced diet. Juicing provides an easy and convenient way to consume various fruits and vegetables, which are rich in vitamins, minerals, and antioxidants essential for maintaining optimal health.

Juicing also offers the advantage of allowing the body to absorb these nutrients better. By extracting the juice from fruits and vegetables, the body can more quickly and efficiently absorb the nutrients than if the foods were eaten whole. This is particularly important for you, who may have compromised digestive systems due to your treatment.

Another benefit of juicing is that it can help reduce inflammation. Chronic inflammation has been linked to various health problems, including cancer. Many fruits and vegetables, such as ginger, turmeric, and leafy greens, contain natural anti-inflammatory compounds that can help reduce inflammation in the body.
In addition to its nutritional benefits, juicing can help detoxify the body. Cancer treatments such as chemotherapy and radiation can generate a lot of toxins in the body, which can hurt overall health. Juicing can help support the body's natural detoxification processes by providing the nutrients needed to eliminate these toxins.

While juicing can benefit cancer patients, it's important to note that not all juices are created equal. Some juices may contain high amounts of sugar or other additives that can harm the body.

It's important to choose fresh, organic produce and avoid adding extra sugars or sweeteners to the juice.

Overall, juicing can be a valuable tool to support your health during treatment. By providing the body with essential nutrients, reducing inflammation, and supporting detoxification processes, juicing can help patients manage their symptoms and improve their overall well-being. Speak to your doctor or a registered dietitian if you have cancer or are caring for someone who does to learn how juicing can be incorporated into your treatment plan.

Chapter 2

Understanding Cancer

Cancer is a complex disease that affects millions of people worldwide. While significant progress has been made in understanding and treating cancer, there is still much to learn. Understanding cancer begins with knowing what it is, how it develops, and the various types of cancer that exist. Now, we will provide an overview of cancer basics, including the various risk factors, stages, and treatment options available. Whether you or a loved one has been diagnosed with cancer or are simply interested in learning more about this complex disease, we will provide valuable insights into the world of cancer and its many challenges.

- **How it Develops**

Cancer is a complex disease that occurs when abnormal cells in the body divide uncontrollably and invade surrounding tissues. The abnormal cells form a tissue mass called a tumour, which can be benign (not cancerous) or malignant (cancerous).

The human body is made up of trillions of cells, which have a specific lifespan and function. During normal cell division, old or damaged cells die and are replaced by new cells. However, in some cases, genetic mutations can occur, causing cells to grow and divide uncontrollably.

These abnormal cells can form a tissue mass, eventually invading surrounding tissues and organs. If left untreated, cancer can spread to other body parts, which is known as metastasis.

There are many types of cancer, each with its own risk factors and treatment options. Some common types of cancer include breast cancer, lung cancer, prostate cancer, skin cancer, and colorectal cancer.

Cancer risk factors include age, family history, lifestyle factors (such as smoking, alcohol consumption, and poor diet), exposure to certain chemicals and radiation, and certain medical conditions.

While there is no guaranteed way to prevent cancer, you can take steps to reduce your risk, such as maintaining a healthy diet and exercise routine, avoiding tobacco and excessive alcohol consumption, and getting regular check-ups and screenings.

Cancer treatment can vary depending on the type and stage of cancer but often includes a combination of surgery, radiation therapy, and chemotherapy. In some cases, complementary therapies such as juicing may help support the body during treatment and promote overall health and well-being.

Working closely with a healthcare provider to develop a personalized treatment plan that meets your individual needs and goals is essential. Regular check-ups and screenings can also help detect cancer early when it is most treatable.

- **Discover the Cancer Types that Can Benefit from this Game-Changing Therapy: Juicing**

Juicing has recently gained popularity as a complementary therapy for cancer treatment. While juicing does not cure cancer, incorporating it into a cancer patient's treatment plan can provide numerous benefits. Certain types of cancer respond better to juicing than others. In this article, we will explore the types of cancer that can be treated with juicing.

1. **Breast cancer:** Breast cancer is the most common cancer in women. Studies have shown that certain nutrients in fruits and vegetables, such as carotenoids, flavonoids, and lignans, may protect against breast cancer. Juicing fruits and vegetables rich in these nutrients, such as kale, spinach, and carrots, can benefit breast cancer patients.

2. **Prostate cancer:** Prostate cancer is the most common cancer in men. Studies have shown that consuming cruciferous vegetables, such as broccoli and cauliflower, can help reduce the risk of prostate cancer. Juicing these vegetables and other vegetables high in antioxidants can provide prostate cancer patients with essential nutrients to support their treatment.

3. **Colorectal cancer:** Colorectal cancer is the second leading cause of cancer-related deaths in the United States. Juicing green leafy vegetables, such as kale and spinach, and beets and carrots, can benefit colorectal cancer patients. These vegetables are high in fiber, which can

help regulate bowel movements and prevent constipation, a common side effect of cancer treatment.

4. **Lung cancer:** Lung cancer is the leading cause of cancer-related deaths worldwide. Antioxidants in fruits and vegetables, such as vitamin C and beta-carotene, have been shown to protect against lung cancer. Juicing fruits and vegetables high in these antioxidants, such as oranges, kale, and carrots, can benefit lung cancer patients.

5. **Pancreatic cancer:** Pancreatic cancer is a rare but deadly form of cancer. Studies have shown that consuming fruits and vegetables high in vitamin C and beta-carotene may help reduce the risk of pancreatic cancer. Juicing fruits and vegetables rich in these nutrients, such as oranges, carrots, and sweet potatoes, can benefit pancreatic cancer patients.

It is important to note that juicing alone cannot treat cancer. Juicing should be used as a complementary therapy and conventional cancer treatments, such as chemotherapy and radiation. It is also essential to consult with a healthcare professional before incorporating juicing into a cancer treatment plan. Certain juices may interact with medications or adversely affect specific cancer types.

In conclusion, incorporating juicing into a cancer treatment plan can benefit cancer patients. Certain types of cancer respond better to juicing than others, and incorporating specific fruits and vegetables into juices can provide essential nutrients to support treatment. Juicing should be used as complementary therapy under a healthcare professional's guidance.

- **The limitations of traditional cancer treatments**

Traditional cancer treatments such as chemotherapy, radiation therapy, and surgery have been the standard of care for many years. While these treatments have been effective in some cases, they also have limitations. In this article, we will explore the limitations of traditional cancer treatments.

Side Effects

One of the major limitations of traditional cancer treatments is the significant side effects that come with them. Chemotherapy, for example, can cause nausea, vomiting, fatigue, and hair loss. Radiation therapy can cause skin irritation and fatigue, while surgery can result in pain, swelling, and limited mobility. These side effects can significantly impact a patient's quality of life and may even lead to treatment discontinuation.

Limited Effectiveness

Another limitation of traditional cancer treatments is their limited effectiveness. While they can be effective in shrinking or removing tumors, they may not be able to eradicate cancer cells; this can lead to cancer returning or becoming resistant to treatment. Additionally, some types of cancer may not respond well to traditional treatments.

Invasive Procedures

Traditional cancer treatments often involve invasive procedures like surgery or radiation therapy. These procedures can be traumatic and may result in long recovery times. In some cases, they may even require the removal of organs, which can significantly impact a patient's quality of life.

Cost

Traditional cancer treatments can also be costly, especially for patients who do not have health insurance. The cost of chemotherapy, radiation therapy, and surgery can increase quickly. It can be a significant financial burden for patients and their families.

Emotional Impact

Finally, traditional cancer treatments can have a significant emotional impact on patients. The physical side effects, combined with the stress of the diagnosis and treatment, can lead to anxiety, depression, and other mental health issues.

Given these limitations, many cancer patients turn to complementary therapies, such as juicing, to support their overall health and well-being. Juicing can provide essential nutrients that boost the immune system and help fight cancer cells. While it should not replace traditional cancer treatments, it can be a valuable addition to a patient's treatment plan.

Chapter 3

Nutrition and Juicing

Nutrition plays a crucial role in our overall health, and this is especially true for cancer patients. Eating a well-balanced diet full of fruits, vegetables, and other nutrient-dense foods can help strengthen the immune system and support the body's natural ability to fight cancer. Juicing is an effective way to ensure that cancer patients get the necessary vitamins, minerals, and antioxidants to support their treatment and recovery. In this section, we will explore the essential nutrients vital for cancer patients and how juicing can provide a convenient and efficient way to incorporate them into their diet.

- **Overview Of Key Nutrients For Cancer Patients**

When fighting cancer, a healthy and balanced diet is crucial. Cancer treatments can often weaken the immune system, making it more difficult for the body to fight infections and diseases. Fortunately, many vital nutrients can help support the immune system and improve overall health during cancer treatment.

The essential nutrients for cancer patients include protein, fiber, healthy fats, vitamins, and minerals. Protein is essential for building and repairing tissue. It is essential for those undergoing chemotherapy, as it can help the body heal after treatment.

Fiber is essential for maintaining a healthy digestive system and can also help regulate blood sugar levels. Healthy fats like those in nuts, seeds, and fatty fish can help improve heart health and reduce inflammation. Vitamins and minerals, such as vitamins D, C, and iron, are also crucial for overall health and immunity.

It's important to note that cancer patients may have unique nutritional needs depending on their type of cancer and the stage of their treatment. Working with a registered dietitian can help ensure they get the proper nutrients in the right amounts to support their overall health and well-being.

- **Unlocking the Power of Juicing for Cancer Treatment**

Juicing can be an essential tool in the fight against cancer for several reasons. First, juicing allows cancer patients to consume a wide range of nutrients in an easily digestible and absorbable form; this is especially important for cancer patients who may have difficulty eating solid foods due to the side effects of treatment.

Juicing supports the immune system by providing the body with the essential vitamins, minerals, and antioxidants to function correctly. Particularly important for defending the body's cells from free radical harm, which is brought on by unstable molecules that can aid in the onset and spread of cancer, antioxidants are essential.

In addition, juicing helps to reduce inflammation, a common side effect of cancer and its treatments. By reducing inflammation, juicing can help improve overall health and reduce the risk of other chronic diseases.

It's important to note that while juicing can be a beneficial addition to a cancer treatment plan, it should not replace traditional medical treatments such as chemotherapy, radiation, and surgery. Juicing should be viewed as a complementary therapy. That can help support overall health and well-being during cancer treatment.

- **The Benefits Of Juicing Over Eating Whole Foods**

Juicing offers several benefits over eating whole foods, especially for cancer patients who may have difficulty consuming solid foods due to the side effects of treatment.

One of the main benefits of juicing is that it allows for the quick and easy consumption of a wide range of nutrients. Juicing can help extract essential vitamins, minerals, and antioxidants from fruits and vegetables, which the body can quickly and easily absorb; this is especially important for cancer patients with weakened digestive systems or difficulty consuming solid foods.

Juicing also offers a way to consume larger quantities of fruits and vegetables than possible by eating whole foods alone; this can be especially important for cancer patients, as many fruits and vegetables contain cancer-fighting compounds and antioxidants essential for supporting the immune system and fighting the disease.

In addition, juicing helps reduce waste, as the pulp and fiber from the fruits and vegetables can be reused in other recipes or composted; this can be especially helpful for cancer patients on a limited budget or who have limited access to fresh produce.

It's important to note that while juicing can offer many benefits over eating whole foods, it should not be viewed as a replacement for a healthy and balanced diet. Whole fruits and vegetables are still essential to a healthy diet, as they provide vital nutrients and fiber that may not be present in juice alone. A balanced nutrition approach, including juicing and whole foods, can provide optimal benefits for cancer patients and support overall health and well-being.

Chapter 4

Juicing Recipes for Optimal Health

Juicing recipes can be an essential addition to a cancer patient's diet, as they offer a quick and easy way to consume a wide range of essential vitamins, minerals, and antioxidants. Juicing can also help reduce inflammation in the body, a common side effect of cancer and its treatments.

In this chapter, we will explore a variety of juicing recipes specifically designed to help support cancer patients. These recipes will include a range of fruits and vegetables that are rich in nutrients and have been shown to have cancer-fighting properties.

These recipes will offer delectable and nourishing choices to support your overall health and well-being while undergoing cancer treatment, whether you're new to juicing or an experienced pro. So grab your juicer and get ready to try out some tasty and beneficial juicing recipes!

- **Juice Your Way to Healing: Powerful Recipes to Beat Cancer, Complete with Ingredients and Preparation Instructions**

Here are three juicing recipes designed to help beat cancer, including a list of ingredients and preparation instructions:

1. Green Machine Juice:

Ingredients:

- 1 cucumber
- 2 stalks of celery
- 1 green apple
- 1 lemon, peeled
- 1 handful of spinach
- 1 handful of kale

Instructions:

1. Wash all of the ingredients thoroughly.
2. Chop the cucumber, celery, and apple into smaller pieces.
3. Add all of the ingredients to your juicer and blend until smooth.
4. Pour the juice into a glass and enjoy immediately.

This juice is packed with cancer-fighting antioxidants and anti-inflammatory compounds from spinach, kale, and lemon. The apple adds a touch of sweetness to balance out the flavors.

2. Carrot and Ginger Juice:

Ingredients:

- 3 large carrots
- 1 inch of fresh ginger
- 1/2 lemon, peeled

Instructions:

1. Wash the carrots and ginger.
2. Peel the lemon.
3. Chop the carrots and ginger into smaller pieces.
4. Add all of the ingredients to your juicer and blend until smooth.
5. Pour the juice into a glass and enjoy immediately.

This juice is high in antioxidants and anti-inflammatory compounds from the carrots and ginger. The lemon adds a zesty flavor that complements the sweetness of the carrots.

3. Berry Blast Juice:

Ingredients:

- 1 cup of mixed berries (blueberries, raspberries, and strawberries)
- 1 green apple
- 1 lemon, peeled
- 1 handful of spinach

Instructions:

1. Wash all of the ingredients thoroughly.
2. Chop the green apple into smaller pieces.
3. Add all of the ingredients to your juicer and blend until smooth.
4. Pour the juice into a glass and enjoy immediately.

This juice is loaded with antioxidants and cancer-fighting compounds from the berries and spinach. The apple adds a touch of sweetness to balance out the tartness of the berries.

These juicing recipes are just a starting point – feel free to experiment with different fruits and vegetables to create your own cancer-fighting juices. And remember, juicing should be part of a balanced diet, so be sure to incorporate whole foods as well to ensure you are getting all the nutrients your body needs to beat cancer.

- **Green Juices**

Green juices have become increasingly popular in recent years, and for good reason. These juices are typically made with a combination of leafy green vegetables and other nutrient-dense ingredients like fruits, herbs, and spices. They are a great way to get a concentrated dose of vitamins, minerals, and antioxidants in a single serving.

When it comes to cancer treatment, green juices can be especially beneficial. Many green vegetables are rich in anti-inflammatory compounds and antioxidants, which can help protect cells from damage and reduce the risk of cancer. Additionally, green juices are often low in sugar and high in fiber, which can help regulate blood sugar levels and support gut health.

Here are some of the most commonly used ingredients in green juices and their potential benefits for cancer patients:

1. **Leafy Greens:** Kale, spinach, collard greens, and other leafy greens are packed with vitamins and minerals like vitamin C, vitamin K, and folate. They also contain antioxidants like beta-carotene and lutein, which can help protect cells from damage and reduce inflammation in the body.
2. **Cruciferous Vegetables:** Vegetables like broccoli, cauliflower, and Brussels sprouts are rich in compounds called glucosinolates, which have been shown to have anti-cancer properties. These vegetables are also high in fiber and vitamin C, which can help support a healthy immune system.
3. **Herbs and Spices:** Ingredients like ginger, turmeric, and mint can add flavor to green juices while also providing additional health benefits. Ginger and turmeric are both potent anti-inflammatory agents, while mint can help soothe the digestive system.
4. **Fruits:** While green juices are primarily made with vegetables, adding a small amount of fruit can help sweeten the juice and make it more palatable. Fruits like apples, pears, and berries are rich in antioxidants and other beneficial nutrients.

Here is a simple recipe for green juice that is perfect for you:

Ingredients:

- 2 cups of spinach
- 1 cup of kale
- 1 cucumber
- 1 green apple
- 1 lemon, peeled
- 1 inch of fresh ginger

Instructions:

1. Wash all of the ingredients thoroughly.
2. Chop the cucumber and apple into smaller pieces.
3. Add all of the ingredients to your juicer and blend until smooth.
4. Pour the juice into a glass and enjoy immediately.

This juice is packed with cancer-fighting nutrients like vitamin C, folate, and beta-carotene. The ginger adds a spicy kick while also providing anti-inflammatory benefits. Plus, it's delicious!

Overall, green juices can be a great way to boost your nutrient intake and support your body's natural cancer-fighting abilities. Just be sure to talk to your doctor before making any significant changes to your diet, especially if you are undergoing cancer treatment.

- **Immune-Boosting Juices**

Immune-boosting juices are an excellent addition to any cancer patient's treatment plan, as they provide a concentrated dose of vitamins and nutrients that can help support the immune system. These juices are typically made with a combination of fruits and vegetables that are high in antioxidants, vitamins, and minerals. Below are some of the best ingredients to include in immune-boosting juices:

1. **Citrus fruits:** Oranges, lemons, limes, and grapefruits are rich in vitamin C, which is essential for a healthy immune system. Vitamin C is a powerful antioxidant that can help protect the body against free radicals and oxidative stress.
2. **Ginger:** Ginger has anti-inflammatory properties and can help support the immune system. It also has a warming effect, which can be comforting for cancer patients.

3. **Turmeric:** Turmeric is another anti-inflammatory ingredient that can help support the immune system. It also contains curcumin, a compound that has been shown to have anticancer properties.
4. **Leafy greens:** Kale, spinach, and other leafy greens are packed with vitamins and minerals that can help support the immune system. They are also high in antioxidants and can help reduce inflammation.
5. **Berries:** Berries such as blueberries, strawberries, and raspberries are high in antioxidants, which can help protect the body against free radicals and oxidative stress.

Here are some immune-boosting juice recipes that you should try:

1. **Citrus and ginger juice:** Combine two oranges, one lemon, one lime, and a small piece of ginger in a juicer. Drink immediately.
2. **Green juice with turmeric:** Combine two handfuls of kale, one cucumber, one apple, one lemon, and one inch of fresh turmeric root in a juicer. Drink immediately.

3. **Berry blast juice:** Combine one cup of mixed berries, one banana, one handful of spinach, and one cup of water in a blender. Blend until smooth, and drink immediately.

When making immune-boosting juices, it's important to choose organic produce whenever possible, as conventionally grown fruits and vegetables may contain pesticides and other harmful chemicals. It's also important to drink the juices immediately after juicing or blending, as the nutrients can degrade quickly.

By incorporating immune-boosting juices into their treatment plan, cancer patients can help support their immune systems and improve their overall health.

- **Anti-Inflammatory Juices**

Anti-inflammatory juices are a great addition to any diet, but they are especially important for those undergoing cancer treatment. Inflammation is a natural response of the immune system to infection or injury. Still, chronic inflammation can contribute to the development and progression of cancer.

Juicing with anti-inflammatory ingredients helps reduce inflammation and support the body's natural healing process.

Here are some of the top anti-inflammatory ingredients to include in your juice recipes:

1. **Turmeric:** This bright yellow spice contains curcumin, a powerful anti-inflammatory compound. Adding turmeric to your juices can help reduce inflammation and support the immune system.
2. **Ginger:** Ginger contains gingerols, which have been shown to have anti-inflammatory effects. Ginger can also help with digestion and nausea, typical side effects of cancer treatment.
3. **Pineapple:** Pineapple contains bromelain, an enzyme with anti-inflammatory properties. It can also help with digestion and is a good source of vitamin C.
4. **Leafy Greens:** Greens such as kale, spinach, and collard greens are packed with anti-inflammatory nutrients like vitamin K, vitamin E, and flavonoids.
5. **Berries:** Like strawberries, blueberries, and raspberries are rich in

anti-inflammatory and antioxidant compounds.

Recipe for an anti-inflammatory juice:

Ingredients:
- 1 cup of kale
- 1 cup of spinach
- 1/2 cup pineapple
- 1/2-inch piece of ginger
- 1/2 lemon, peeled
- 1/2 cup berries (blueberries or strawberries)

Instructions:
1. Wash all ingredients thoroughly.
2. Put all the ingredients in a juicer and juice.
3. Serve immediately and enjoy.

Incorporating anti-inflammatory juices into your diet can be a great way to support your body during cancer treatment.

- **Antioxidant-Rich Juices**

Antioxidants are a group of compounds that help protect cells from damage caused by free radicals, which are unstable molecules produced during normal cellular metabolism and exposure to environmental factors such as pollution and radiation. Antioxidants are essential for cancer patients because they can help support the immune system and reduce oxidative stress, which has been linked to the development and progression of cancer.

Juicing with antioxidant-rich ingredients can help boost the body's antioxidant levels and support overall health. Here are some of the top antioxidant-rich ingredients to include in your juice recipes:

1. **Berries:** Berries such as blueberries, raspberries, and strawberries are some of the richest sources of antioxidants, including anthocyanins, flavonols, and vitamin C.
2. **Citrus fruits:** Citrus fruits like oranges, lemons, and grapefruits are rich in vitamin C, a powerful antioxidant that can help boost the immune system.
3. **Carrots:** Carrots are rich in beta-carotene, which is converted to vitamin A in the body and acts as an antioxidant.
4. **Green tea:** Green tea contains polyphenols, including EGCG, which have been shown to have antioxidant and anti-cancer properties.

5. **Turmeric**: Turmeric contains curcumin, a powerful antioxidant and anti-inflammatory compound.

Here is a recipe for an antioxidant-rich juice:
Ingredients:

- 1 cup mixed berries (blueberries, raspberries, and strawberries)
- 1 orange, peeled
- 1 carrot, peeled
- 1/2-inch piece of ginger
- 1 green tea bag, steeped and cooled

Instructions:
1. Wash all ingredients thoroughly.
2. Add berries, orange, carrot, and ginger to a juicer and juice.
3. Add cooled green tea to the juice and stir.
4. Serve immediately and enjoy.

Incorporating antioxidant-rich juices into your diet can significantly support overall health and well-being during cancer treatment.

- **Detoxifying Juices**

Detoxifying juices are a great way to support the body's natural detoxification processes and promote overall health. These juices are typically made with ingredients rich in antioxidants, vitamins, and minerals that help eliminate toxins from the body while also boosting the immune system and reducing inflammation.

Here are the best detoxifying juices that will help you cleanse your body and improve your overall health:

1. **Green Detox Juice:** This juice is made with kale, spinach, cucumber, celery, lemon, and ginger. These ingredients are all rich in antioxidants and vitamins that help detoxify the body and support the immune system.
2. **Beetroot and Carrot Juice:** Beetroots are high in antioxidants and are known for their detoxifying properties. Carrots are rich in vitamin A, which supports healthy skin and eyesight. This juice is a great way to detoxify the liver and support overall health.
3. **Citrus Detox Juice:** This juice is made with grapefruit, lemon, lime, and orange. Citrus fruits are high in vitamin C, which supports the immune system and helps to eliminate toxins from the body. This juice

is also a great source of electrolytes, which can help to keep you hydrated.

4. **Pineapple and Ginger Juice:** Pineapple contains an enzyme called bromelain, which supports healthy digestion and helps to reduce inflammation in the body. Ginger is a natural anti-inflammatory and can help reduce nausea and support healthy digestion. This juice is a great way to support overall health and detoxify the body.

5. **Cucumber and Mint Juice:** Cucumbers are high in water content, which can help flush out toxins from the body. Mint is a natural digestive aid that can help reduce inflammation. This juice is a refreshing way to support the body's natural detoxification processes.

When making detoxifying juices, using fresh, organic ingredients is essential whenever possible. It's also important to consume these juices as part of a healthy and balanced diet and to stay hydrated by drinking plenty of water throughout the day. Incorporating these juices into your diet can support your body's natural detoxification processes and improve overall health and well-being.

Chapter 5

The Cancer-Fighting Juice: 150 Must-Try Recipes

- **Mouthwatering Recipes**

1. Green Machine: kale, cucumber, celery, apple, lemon, ginger
2. Citrus Sunrise: oranges, grapefruit, carrots, turmeric, cayenne pepper
3. Pink Lady: beets, strawberries, apples, ginger, lemon
4. Golden Glow: carrots, sweet potato, pineapple, ginger
5. Spicy Tomato: tomatoes, celery, cucumber, jalapeño, lemon
6. Tropical Paradise: mango, pineapple, papaya, coconut water
7. Cucumber Mint: cucumber, mint, lemon, honey
8. Carrot Turmeric: carrots, turmeric, ginger, and orange
9. Kale Yeah: kale, spinach, cucumber,

celery, apple, lemon
10. Blueberry Basil: blueberries, basil, apple, lemon, honey
11. Pomegranate Power: pomegranate, kale, ginger, and lemon
12. Sweet Greens: kale, apple, cucumber, lemon, honey
13. Orange Creamsicle: oranges, carrots, vanilla protein powder, almond milk
14. Beet It: beets, cucumber, ginger, lemon, honey
15. Watermelon Cooler: watermelon, mint, lime
16. Green Lemonade: spinach, cucumber, apple, and lemon
17. Spicy Green: kale, celery, green apple, jalapeño, lime
18. Berry Beet: beets, raspberries, blueberries, apples, lemon
19. Carrot Pineapple: carrots, pineapple, ginger, and lemon
20. Turmeric Tonic: turmeric, ginger, lemon, honey
21. Melon Medley: honeydew, cantaloupe, cucumber, mint
22. Orange Carrot Ginger: oranges, carrots, ginger, lemon
23. Royal Nectar: A mix of golden kiwi,

pineapple, and turmeric for a sweet, anti-inflammatory drink that supports immune function and fights cancer.

24. Carrot Cucumber Ginger: carrots, cucumber, ginger, lemon
25. Green Tea Infusion: green tea, spinach, cucumber, honey
26. Mango Tango: mango, orange, apple, ginger
27. Spicy Pineapple: pineapple, ginger, jalapeño, lemon
28. Red Recovery: beets, carrots, apple, lemon, ginger
29. Cucumber Limeade: cucumber, lime, honey
30. Tropical Turmeric: pineapple, mango, turmeric, ginger
31. Carrot Apple Ginger: carrots, apple, ginger, lemon
32. Berry Boost: blueberries, strawberries, raspberries, almond milk
33. Green Machine 2.0: kale, cucumber, celery, green apple, lemon, parsley
34. Ginger Lemon Blast: ginger, lemon, and honey
35. Apple Cider Vinegar Tonic: apple cider vinegar, lemon, honey, cinnamon
36. Pineapple Cucumber Mint: pineapple,

cucumber, mint, and lemon

37. Carrot Orange Pineapple: carrots, orange, pineapple, ginger
38. Ginger Peach: peaches, ginger, lemon
39. Beet Berry Basil: beets, raspberries, blueberries, basil, and lemon
40. Green Detox: kale, spinach, cucumber, celery, green apple, lemon
41. Spicy Apple: apples, jalapeño, lime, honey
42. Watermelon Lime Mint: watermelon, lime, mint.
43. Carrot Ginger Lime: carrots, ginger, lime
44. Golden Elixir: A blend of turmeric, ginger, carrot, and orange to boost immunity and reduce inflammation.
45. Berry Blast: A mix of strawberries, blueberries, raspberries, and spinach for a powerful antioxidant boost.
46. Sunset Serenade: A delicious blend of grapefruit, orange, and carrot, rich in vitamin C and beta-carotene.
47. Green Monster: A mix of kale, cucumber, celery, and green apple for a nutrient-dense and alkalizing juice.
48. Sweet & Spicy: A blend of sweet potato, carrot, ginger, and cinnamon to regulate blood sugar levels and reduce

inflammation.

49. Lemon-Lime Refresher: A mix of lemon, lime, cucumber, and mint to aid digestion and support liver function.

50. Purple Reign: A blend of beets, blueberries, and kale, rich in antioxidants and anti-inflammatory compounds

51. Pineapple Paradise: A pineapple, ginger, and turmeric mix to aid digestion and reduce inflammation.

52. Carrot Cake Delight: A blend of carrot, apple, cinnamon, and nutmeg for a tasty and nutritious treat.

53. Sunshine in a Glass: A mix of orange, grapefruit, and lemon to boost immunity and provide a dose of vitamin C

54. Radiant Recovery: A blend of kale, cucumber, celery, green apple, lemon, ginger, and turmeric for a powerful antioxidant and anti-inflammatory boost.

55. Immune Elixir: A mix of grapefruit, orange, lemon, and ginger to support immune function and reduce inflammation.

56. Pink Power: A blend of beets, strawberries, and watermelon for a high dose of antioxidants and anti-inflammatory compounds

57. Turmeric Tonic: A mix of turmeric, ginger, lemon, and honey for a powerful anti-inflammatory and immune-boosting blend.

58. Berry Beet Blast: A combination of beets, raspberries, blueberries, and spinach for a powerful antioxidant boost.

59. Carrot Ginger Sunrise: A mix of carrots, ginger, orange, and lemon for a refreshing and immune-boosting blend.

60. Green Goddess: A blend of kale, spinach, cucumber, celery, green apple, and lemon for a nutrient-dense and alkalizing juice.

61. Orange Blossom: A mix of oranges, carrots, and ginger for a delicious and nutritious blend.

62. Spicy Carrot Ginger: A mix of carrots, ginger, jalapeno, and lemon for a spicy and immune-boosting blend.

63. Blueberry Basil Bliss: A combination of blueberries, basil, lemon, and honey for a refreshing and antioxidant-rich blend

64. Mango Tango Twist: A blend of mango, orange, pineapple, and coconut water for a delicious and immune-boosting juice.

65. Pineapple Cucumber Mint: A mix of pineapple, cucumber, mint, and lemon for a refreshing and antioxidant-rich blend

66. Ginger Peach Punch: A blend of peaches, ginger, and lemon for a refreshing and immune-boosting blend

67. Acai Berry Blast: A mix of acai berries, blueberries, raspberries, and almond milk for a powerful antioxidant and anti-inflammatory blend

68. Grapefruit Ginger Zinger: A combination of grapefruit, ginger, lemon, and honey for a zesty and immune-boosting blend

69. Cucumber Lemon Cooler: A cucumber, lemon, and honey mix for a refreshing and immune-boosting blend

70. Kiwi Kale Crush: A blend of kiwi, kale, green apple, and lemon for a nutrient-dense and immune-boosting juice.

71. Orange Ginger Spice: A mix of oranges, ginger, cinnamon, and honey for a spicy and immune-boosting blend

72. Strawberry Basil Sipper: A combination of strawberries, basil, and lemon for a refreshing and antioxidant-rich blend

73. Lemon Lime Refresher: A mix of lemon, lime, cucumber, and mint to aid digestion and support liver function.

74. Apple Cider Vinegar Tonic: A blend of apple cider vinegar, lemon, honey, and

cinnamon for a powerful
immune-boosting and anti-inflammatory
blend.

75. Beet Berry Basil Blast: A mix of beets,
raspberries, blueberries, basil, and lemon
for a powerful antioxidant and
anti-inflammatory boost.

76. Carrot Orange Pineapple Perfection: A
combination of carrots, orange, pineapple,
and ginger for a delicious and
immune-boosting blend.

77. Ginger Lemon Detox: A mix of ginger,
lemon, and honey for a powerful
immune-boosting and detoxifying blend.

78. Watermelon Mint Cooler: A combination
of watermelon, mint, and lime for a
refreshing and immune-boosting blend.

79. Carrot Ginger Limeade: A blend of
carrots, ginger, lime, and honey for a zesty
and immune-boosting juice.

80. Golden Elixir: A mix of turmeric, ginger,
carrot, and orange creates a powerful
anti-inflammatory and immune-boosting
blend.

81. Golden Sunrise: A blend of carrots,
oranges, ginger, and turmeric for a potent
anti-inflammatory and immune-boosting
juice.

82. Sweet Greens: A mix of spinach, kale, green apple, cucumber, and pear for a sweet and nutritious green juice.

83. Red Radiance: A blend of beets, strawberries, and watermelon for a juice rich in antioxidants and anti-inflammatory compounds.

84. Citrus Zing: A mix of grapefruit, lemon, lime, and ginger for a tangy and refreshing juice that aids in digestion.

85. Berry Beet Blast: A mix of beets, blueberries, raspberries, and strawberries for a juice packed with antioxidants and cancer-fighting properties.

86. Mango Tango: A mango, ginger, and turmeric blend for tropical and anti-inflammatory juice.

87. Pink Power: A mix of watermelon, raspberries, and mint for a refreshing, hydrating juice rich in antioxidants.

88. Carrot Topper: A mix of carrots, celery, and apple for a sweet and nutritious juice that supports liver and kidney function

89. Sweet and Sour: A blend of pineapple, lemon, and ginger for a sweet and tangy juice that aids digestion and reduces inflammation.

90. Green Glow: A mix of spinach,

cucumber, celery, green apple, and lemon for a nutrient-dense and alkalizing juice that promotes detoxification.

91.● Purple Passion: A blend of blueberries, blackberries, strawberries, and raspberries for a juice rich in antioxidants and cancer-fighting properties

92.● Kiwi Kiss: A mix of kiwi, lime, and honey for a refreshing and immune-boosting juice that supports healthy digestion and aids in nutrient absorption.

93.● Red Reboot: A blend of beets, carrots, ginger, and lemon for a juice that promotes liver function and reduces inflammation.

94. Carrot Craze: A mix of carrots, oranges, and ginger for a sweet and spicy juice that supports healthy digestion and immune function

95. Tropical Twist: A pineapple, mango, and papaya blend for a tropical and anti-inflammatory juice rich in enzymes and vitamins.

96. Berry Beautiful: A mix of strawberries, raspberries, blackberries, and mint for a refreshing and antioxidant-rich juice that supports healthy skin and digestion

97. Lemon Limeade: A mix of lemon, lime, honey, and water for a refreshing and alkalizing juice that supports detoxification and digestion

98. Grapefruit Ginger: A blend of grapefruit, ginger, and honey for a tangy and anti-inflammatory juice that supports immune function

99. Orange Oasis: A mix of oranges, carrots, and turmeric for a refreshing and immune-boosting juice that supports healthy skin and digestion

100. Kale Crush: A blend of kale, cucumber, celery, and lemon for a nutrient-dense and alkalizing juice that supports detoxification and digestion.

101. Red Rejuvenator: A mix of beets, strawberries, and ginger for a juice rich in antioxidants and anti-inflammatory compounds that promotes healthy blood flow.

102. Sweet Sunshine: A blend of carrots, oranges, and pineapple for a sweet and tangy juice that supports healthy digestion and immune function

103. Cucumber Cooler: A mix of cucumber, lime, and mint for a refreshing, hydrating juice that supports healthy skin and

digestion

104. Ginger Green: A blend of spinach, kale, green apple, ginger, and lemon for a nutrient-dense and anti-inflammatory juice that supports healthy digestion and immune function

105. Purple Powerhouse: A mix of blueberries, blackberries, raspberries, and kale for a juice rich in antioxidants and anti-inflammatory compounds that promotes healthy brain function and helps fight against cancer.

106. Immunity Booster: A blend of kiwi, lemon, orange, and spinach to strengthen the immune system and fight off cancer cells

107. Spicy Green: A mix of green apple, cucumber, jalapeno, and cilantro to reduce inflammation and provide a kick of heat

108. Purple Love: A blend of purple cabbage, blackberries, and ginger for a powerful antioxidant boost.

109. Citrus Splash: A mix of grapefruit, lime, lemon, and mint to aid in digestion and provide a dose of vitamin C

110. Orange Creamsicle: A blend of orange, vanilla, and coconut milk for a creamy and delicious treat high in antioxidants

111.   Green Goddess: A mix of kale, parsley, celery, and pear to detoxify the body and provide a nutrient-dense juice

112.   Beet It: A blend of beets, carrots, and ginger to reduce inflammation and provide a dose of vitamins and minerals

113.   Melon Medley: A mix of watermelon, honeydew, and mint for a refreshing and hydrating juice that is also high in antioxidants

114.   Lemon Ginger Zing: A blend of lemon, ginger, and apple cider vinegar to aid in digestion and reduce inflammation

115.   Turmeric Tango: A turmeric, orange, and pineapple mix to reduce inflammation and boost antioxidants

116.   Immune Boost: A blend of orange, ginger, and turmeric to support the immune system and reduce inflammation

117.   Sunset Glow: A mix of carrot, grapefruit, and ginger for a delicious and nutritious juice

118.   Purple Haze: A blend of blueberries, raspberries, and kale, rich in antioxidants and anti-inflammatory compounds

119.   The Ultimate Detox: A mix of cucumber, celery, kale, and lemon for a powerful detoxifying juice.

120. Pineapple Ginger Blast: A mix of pineapple, ginger, and mint to aid digestion and reduce inflammation.
121. Lemon Berry Blast: A blend of lemon, blueberries, and strawberries for a refreshing and immune-boosting juice
122. Turmeric Tonic: A mix of turmeric, ginger, and lemon for a powerful anti-inflammatory and immune-boosting juice
123. Berry Beet Blast: A blend of beets, raspberries, and blueberries for a delicious and nutrient-packed juice
124. Minty Melon: A mix of watermelon, mint, and lime for a refreshing and hydrating juice
125. Green Goddess: A blend of spinach, cucumber, celery, green apple, and lemon for a nutrient-dense and alkalizing juice
126. Sunrise Bliss: A blend of oranges, carrots, and turmeric for a powerful dose of vitamin C and anti-inflammatory benefits
127. Ginger Lime Cooler: A mix of ginger, lime, and cucumber for a refreshing and invigorating drink that aids digestion and reduces inflammation
128. Ruby Red Rejuvenator: A combination

of beets, strawberries, and raspberries for a high-antioxidant drink that helps to cleanse the blood and support the immune system

129.   Pineapple Green Goddess: A mix of pineapple, kale, and cucumber makes a sweet and refreshing drink rich in nutrients and helps to alkalize the body.

130.   Minty Melon Medley: A blend of watermelon, honeydew, and mint for a hydrating and cooling drink that supports the immune system and aids digestion

131.   Pineapple Green Goddess: A mix of pineapple, kale, and cucumber for a sweet and refreshing drink that is rich in nutrients and helps to alkalize the body.

132.   Spicy Carrot Kick: A mix of carrots, ginger, and cayenne pepper for a spicy and energizing drink that helps to reduce inflammation and boost the metabolism

133.   Cherry Berry Blast: A combination of cherries, blueberries, and raspberries for a delicious and antioxidant-rich drink that supports the immune system and helps to fight cancer

134.   Green Tea Infusion: A blend of green tea, lemon, and honey for a refreshing and antioxidant-rich drink that helps to reduce

inflammation and support the immune
system.

135.   Turmeric Sunshine: A mix of turmeric,
oranges, and carrots for a sunny and
anti-inflammatory drink that helps to
boost the immune system and fight cancer

136.   Golden Carrot Elixir: A combination
of carrots, apples, and turmeric for a sweet
and spicy drink that is rich in antioxidants
and helps to reduce inflammation.

137.   Radiant Glow: A mix of carrots,
oranges, and ginger for a high-vitamin C
drink that supports healthy skin and boosts
the immune system.

138.   Sunset Serenity: A combination of
papaya, oranges, and turmeric for a
refreshing, immune-boosting drink that
helps reduce inflammation.

139.   Emerald Elixir: A mix of cucumber,
spinach, green apple, and lime for a
hydrating and alkalizing drink that
supports overall health and well-being.

140.   Citrus Zinger: A mix of grapefruit,
lemon, and ginger for a tart and tangy
drink high in vitamin C and
anti-inflammatory compounds.

141.   Garden Goddess: A combination of
kale, cucumber, celery, green apple, and

lemon for a nutrient-packed and alkalizing drink that supports overall health and well-being.

142. Cherry Crush: A mix of cherries, pomegranate, and ginger for a delicious and antioxidant-rich drink that supports the immune system and helps to reduce inflammation.

143. Beet the Odds: A combination of beets, carrots, and apples for a high-nitrate drink that helps to lower blood pressure and supports overall cardiovascular health.

144. Pineapple Ginger Zest: A mix of pineapple, ginger, and lime for a refreshing and energizing drink that supports digestion and reduces inflammation.

145. Blueberry Bliss: A blend of blueberries, strawberries, and raspberries for a delicious and high-antioxidant drink that supports the immune system and helps to fight against cancer.

146. Topaz Tonic: A combination of green apple, cucumber, lemon, and ginger for a refreshing and detoxifying drink that supports liver function and overall well-being.

147. Aquamarine Elixir: A mix of

pineapple, cucumber, and mint for a hydrating and anti-inflammatory drink that supports digestive health and overall wellness.

148.   Opal Oasis: A blend of watermelon, lime, and basil for a refreshing and hydrating drink that supports immune function and helps to reduce inflammation.

149.   Turquoise Temptation: A combination of kale, blueberries, and ginger for a high-antioxidant and anti-inflammatory drink that supports brain health and helps to fight against cancer.

150.   Emerald Empowerment: A mix of spinach, green apple, celery, and lemon for a nutrient-dense and alkalizing drink that supports overall health and well-being.

- **Green Machine: kale, cucumber, celery, apple, lemon, ginger**

Green Machine is a refreshing and nutrient-packed juice. The star ingredient Kale is rich in antioxidants, anti-inflammatory compounds, and cancer-fighting phytochemicals. Cucumbers and celery provide hydration and additional vitamins and minerals, while apples and lemons add sweetness and tang. Ginger, a powerful anti-inflammatory and immune booster, adds a zingy kick to this delicious juice.

Ingredients:

- 2 cups kale leaves
- 1 medium cucumber
- 4 celery stalks
- 1 green apple
- 1/2 lemon, peeled
- 1-inch piece of ginger

Directions:

1. Wash all ingredients thoroughly.
2. Chop the kale leaves into small pieces.
3. Cut the cucumber, celery, and apple into chunks.
4. Peel the lemon.
5. Peel the ginger and chop it into small pieces.
6. Add all ingredients into a juicer, starting with the kale leaves and ending with the ginger.
7. Stir the juice and serve over ice.

8. Enjoy the refreshing and nutrient-packed Green Machine juice!

- **Citrus Sunrise: oranges, grapefruit, carrots, turmeric, cayenne pepper**

Citrus Sunrise is a delicious and refreshing juice that is perfect for cancer patients who want to boost their immune system and fight inflammation. Oranges and grapefruits are rich in vitamin C, which is an essential nutrient for immune system health. Carrots are packed with beta-carotene, which is converted to vitamin A in the body and plays a role in immune function. Turmeric contains curcumin, a powerful anti-inflammatory compound that has been shown to inhibit the growth of cancer cells. Cayenne pepper contains capsaicin, which can reduce pain and inflammation and also has cancer-fighting properties.

To make Citrus Sunrise, you will need:

- 2 oranges, peeled
- 1 grapefruit, peeled
- 3 carrots, peeled
- 1-inch piece of turmeric root, peeled

- 1/4 teaspoon cayenne pepper

Simply juice all of the ingredients together and enjoy immediately. This juice is best consumed in the morning to kickstart your day and provide a burst of energy. It can also be a great pre-workout drink due to its energizing and anti-inflammatory properties. So, why not give Citrus Sunrise a try and experience its health benefits for yourself?

- **Pink Lady: beets, strawberries, apples, ginger, lemon**

Pink Lady Juice Recipe:

Ingredients:

- 1 medium-sized beetroot, peeled and sliced
- 1 cup of strawberries
- 2 green apples, cored and sliced
- 1-inch pieces of fresh ginger, peeled and sliced
- 1 lemon, peeled and sliced

Instructions:

1. Prepare all the ingredients by washing, peeling, and slicing them.
2. Run all the ingredients through a juicer, one at a time, and collect the juice in a glass.
3. Stir the juice well and serve immediately.

Benefits:

The Pink Lady juice is loaded with antioxidants, vitamins, and minerals that are beneficial for cancer patients. Beetroot is high in betalains, which have been found to have anti-inflammatory and antioxidant properties.

Strawberries are rich in Vitamin C, which boosts the immune system and helps fight cancer cells. Green apples are a good source of dietary fiber and antioxidants, and they are also known to help reduce the risk of developing colon cancer. Ginger has anti-inflammatory and antioxidant properties and is known to help reduce nausea and vomiting that can be caused by chemotherapy.

Finally, lemon is high in Vitamin C and citric acid, which can help improve digestion and boost the immune system.

- **Golden Glow: carrots, sweet potato, pineapple, ginger**

Golden Glow Juice Recipe:

Ingredients:

- 2 medium carrots
- 1 small sweet potato
- 1 cup pineapple chunks
- 1-inch piece of fresh ginger

Instructions:

1. Wash and prepare all ingredients.
2. Cut the carrots and sweet potato into small pieces to fit through the juicer.
3. Juice the carrots, sweet potato, pineapple, and ginger together.
4. Stir the juice well before serving.
5. Pour over ice and enjoy!

Benefits:

The Golden Glow juice is a nutrient-dense and delicious way to get a boost of antioxidants, vitamins, and minerals. Carrots and sweet potatoes are excellent sources of beta-carotene, which is converted to vitamin A in the body and helps support healthy skin and vision. Pineapple is rich in vitamin C, which helps support the immune system and contains bromelain, an enzyme with anti-inflammatory properties.

Ginger has anti-inflammatory and antioxidant properties and may help relieve digestive discomfort. This juice is perfect for cancer patients looking to support their overall health and well-being.

- **Spicy Tomato: tomatoes, celery, cucumber, jalapeño, lemon**

Spicy Tomato is a perfect blend of juicy tomatoes, refreshing cucumber, and crunchy celery with a spicy kick of jalapeño and a zing of lemon. This recipe is not only delicious but also packed with essential nutrients that can boost the immune system and fight cancer.

Ingredients:

- 4 medium-sized tomatoes
- 2 stalks of celery
- 1 small cucumber
- 1 small jalapeño pepper

- 1 lemon, peeled
- 1/4 teaspoon sea salt
- 1/4 teaspoon black pepper

Instructions:

1. Wash all the ingredients thoroughly.
2. Cut the tomatoes, celery, and cucumber into small pieces.
3. Remove the seeds and stem from the jalapeño pepper, and cut it into small pieces.
4. Juice all the ingredients in a juicer.
5. Stir the sea salt and black pepper into the juice.
6. Pour the juice into a glass and serve immediately.

This Spicy Tomato juice is a great source of vitamin C, potassium, and lycopene, a powerful antioxidant that has been shown to have anti-cancer properties. It also contains capsaicin, a compound found in spicy foods like jalapeño pepper, which has been found to have anti-inflammatory and anti-tumor properties.

If you prefer a milder taste, you can remove the seeds and white membrane from the jalapeño pepper before juicing. This recipe can also be adjusted to fit individual preferences by adding more or less jalapeño pepper and adjusting the seasoning to taste.

Overall, Spicy Tomato juice is a delicious and nutritious way to incorporate cancer-fighting ingredients into your diet.

- **Tropical Paradise: mango, pineapple, papaya, coconut water**

With just one sip of Tropical Paradise's delicious and energizing juice, you'll be whisked away to a tropical island. In addition to being a great way to quench your thirst, this juice offers a variety of nutrients that are good for your health, especially if you are fighting cancer.

Mangoes are a great source of antioxidants, vitamin C, and beta-carotene, essential for supporting the immune system and fighting off cancer cells. Bromelain, an enzyme found in pineapples with anti-inflammatory and digestive benefits, is also found in pineapples.

Papaya is rich in antioxidants, vitamin C, and folate, which can help prevent cellular damage and promote healthy cell growth. Electrolytes, which are essential for preserving hydration and supporting healthy kidney function, are found naturally in coconut water.

One mango, one cup of pineapple, one cup of papaya, and one cup of coconut water should be blended to make this juice. Serve over ice and enjoy your tropical paradise in a glass.

- **Cucumber Mint: cucumber, mint, lemon, honey**

Cucumber mint juice is a cooling and hydrating juice for hot summer days. It is not only delectable but also has a lot of health advantages. The antioxidant content of cucumbers is high, and they also contain potassium, magnesium, and vitamins A, C, and K. Mint is well known for its calming effects and ability to aid digestion. While honey adds a hint of sweetness, lemon adds a burst of vitamin C.

Ingredients:

- 2 cucumbers
- A handful of fresh mint leaves
- 1 lemon, peeled
- 1-2 teaspoons of honey (optional)

Instructions:

1. Wash and chop the cucumbers, leaving the skin on.
2. Remove the leaves from the mint stems.
3. Peel the lemon.
4. Add the cucumbers, mint leaves, and lemon to a juicer and juice.
5. If desired, add honey to taste.
6. Stir the juice and pour it into a glass.
7. Serve chilled or over ice.

This Cucumber Mint juice is not only delicious, but it is also a great way to hydrate and nourish your body. It is a perfect drink for anyone looking for a refreshing and healthy beverage.

- **Carrot Turmeric: carrots, turmeric, ginger, and orange**

Carrot Turmeric is a delicious and nutritious juicing recipe that can help cancer patients with its anti-inflammatory properties. Here's how to make it:

Ingredients:

- 4 large carrots
- 1-inch piece of fresh turmeric root
- 1-inch of fresh ginger root
- 1 large orange

Preparation:

1. Wash the carrots, turmeric, and ginger thoroughly.
2. Cut off the ends of the carrots and slice them into smaller pieces.
3. Peel the turmeric and ginger roots and cut them into smaller pieces.
4. Peel the orange and remove the seeds.
5. Put all the ingredients through a juicer.
6. Stir the juice well and pour it into a glass.
7. Serve immediately.

To strengthen your immune system, reduce inflammation, and advance general health, this recipe contains antioxidants, vitamins, and minerals. Carrots, turmeric, and ginger together have anti-inflammatory properties. In addition, the orange provides more vitamin C and a hint of sweetness. Give this recipe a try to help support your cancer treatment plan.

- **Kale Yeah: kale, spinach, cucumber, celery, apple, lemon**

Recipe for "Kale Yeah":

Ingredients:

- 1 bunch of kale
- 1 handful of spinach
- 1 cucumber
- 2 celery stalks
- 1 green apple
- 1 lemon

Instructions:

1. Wash all produce thoroughly.
2. Remove stems from kale and spinach.
3. Cut cucumber and apple into chunks.
4. Juice all ingredients together, starting with the kale and ending with the lemon.
5. Stir the juice and pour it into a glass.
6. Serve immediately and enjoy!

This juice contains nutrients and antioxidants from kale, spinach, cucumber, celery, apple, and lemon. It's a wonderful way to begin your day and increase your body's nutrition and energy levels. The apple's sweetness and the lemon's sourness balance the greens' flavors, making for a delectable and energizing juice.

- **Blueberry Basil: blueberries, basil, apple, lemon, honey**

Blueberry Basil Juice Recipe:

Ingredients:

- 1 cup of fresh blueberries
- 5-6 large basil leaves
- 2 green apples
- 1 lemon
- 1 teaspoon of honey (optional)

Instructions:

1. Wash all the ingredients thoroughly and chop them into small pieces.
2. Add the blueberries, basil leaves, and chopped apples into the juicer.
3. Squeeze the juice from the lemon and pour it into the juicer.

4. Mix well and add honey if desired.
5. Serve chilled.

Benefits:

This juice is packed with antioxidants and anti-inflammatory compounds. Anthocyanins, which are abundant in blueberries and have been shown to lower the risk of cancer. Basil is renowned for having anti-inflammatory qualities that can help lower stress. Apples are a good source of fiber and lemons up the vitamin C content. This juice will help you start the day off right and will strengthen your immune system.

- **Pomegranate Power: pomegranate, kale, ginger, and lemon**

Here's a recipe for Pomegranate Power:

Ingredients:

- 1 cup pomegranate seeds
- 2 cups of kale
- 1-inch piece of ginger, peeled
- 1 lemon, peeled
- 1 apple, cored

Instructions:

1. Wash and chop all ingredients.
2. Add ingredients to your juicer and juice.
3. Pour the juice into a glass and enjoy.

This juice is packed with nutrients and antioxidants from the pomegranate and kale, while the ginger adds a spicy kick and the lemon and apple provide a touch of sweetness. It's a great way to boost your energy and support your immune system while undergoing cancer treatment.

- **Sweet Greens: kale, apple, cucumber, lemon, honey**

Ingredients:

- 2 cups of kale leaves
- 1 green apple
- 1 cucumber
- 1/2 lemon, juiced
- 1 tablespoon honey

Instructions:

1. Rinse all the ingredients thoroughly.
2. Cut the apple and cucumber into small pieces.

3. Place all the ingredients in a juicer and extract the juice.
4. Stir in the honey.
5. Serve and enjoy.

Benefits:

- Kale is a nutrient-dense leafy green that is rich in antioxidants, vitamins, and minerals.
- Green apples are a great source of fiber and vitamin C.
- Cucumbers are low in calories and high in water content, making them great for hydration.
- Lemons are high in vitamin C and have anti-inflammatory properties.
- Honey is a natural sweetener that has antioxidant and anti-inflammatory properties.

This juice is a great way to incorporate nutrient-dense greens into your diet while still satisfying your sweet tooth. The addition of honey provides natural sweetness without the need for processed sugar. The high water content of the cucumber and the hydrating properties of the lemon make this juice a refreshing and energizing option.

- **Orange Creamsicle: oranges, carrots, vanilla protein powder, almond milk**

Orange Creamsicle Juice Recipe:

Ingredients:

- 3 oranges, peeled
- 3 large carrots, peeled
- 1 scoop of vanilla protein powder
- 1/2 cup unsweetened almond milk

Instructions:

1. Cut the oranges and carrots into smaller pieces to fit in your juicer.
2. Juice the oranges and carrots together.
3. In a separate blender, combine the orange carrot juice, vanilla protein powder, and almond milk.
4. Blend on high speed until the mixture is smooth and creamy.
5. Pour into a glass and serve immediately.

Benefits:

- Oranges are a great source of vitamin C, which can boost the immune system.
- Carrots are rich in beta-carotene, an antioxidant that may help protect against cancer.
- Vanilla protein powder can provide additional protein, which is important for tissue repair and maintenance during cancer treatment.
- Almond milk is a dairy-free alternative to milk that is low in calories and may help reduce inflammation.

This juice is a great option for cancer patients experiencing taste changes or difficulty eating solid foods. It is easy to swallow and has a sweet, creamy flavor reminiscent of a classic creamsicle. The added protein and vitamins from the powder and almond milk can also provide additional nutrition to support the body during treatment.

- **Beet It: beets, cucumber, ginger, lemon, honey**

Ingredients:

- 1 medium beet, peeled and chopped
- 1 cucumber, peeled and chopped

- 1-inch piece of ginger, peeled and grated
- 1 lemon, juiced
- 1 teaspoon honey

Instructions:

1. Wash and prep all the ingredients.
2. Start with the beet, then add the cucumber, ginger, and lemon before putting them all through a juicer.
3. Mix in the honey and stir well.
4. Serve over ice and enjoy!

Benefits:

This juice is high in antioxidants and anti-inflammatory compounds due to the presence of beets, which also help detoxify the body. Cucumber adds hydration and helps reduce inflammation.

Ginger adds a spicy kick and is known for its anti-nausea properties, making it helpful for cancer patients undergoing chemotherapy. Lemon juice helps boost immunity and provides vitamin C. Honey adds natural sweetness and has antibacterial and antiviral properties.

- **Watermelon Cooler: watermelon, mint, lime**

Watermelon Cooler Recipe:

Ingredients:

- 4 cups of chopped watermelon
- 1/4 cup of fresh mint leaves
- 1 lime, juiced
- 1 cup of ice

Instructions:

1. Place the chopped watermelon, mint leaves, and lime juice into a blender.
2. Blend on high until smooth.
3. Add the ice and blend again until the ice is crushed and the mixture is well combined.
4. Pour the juice into a glass and enjoy.

This refreshing and hydrating juice is perfect for a hot summer day. Lycopene, an antioxidant that helps prevent cancer, is present in watermelon and contributes to its high water content. Mint leaves add a fresh flavor and also aid in digestion. Vitamin C, which supports the immune system, is abundant in lime juice and gives it a tangy zing.

- **Green Lemonade: spinach, cucumber, apple, and lemon**

Ingredients:

- 2 cups of spinach
- 1 medium cucumber, sliced
- 1 green apple, sliced
- 1 lemon, juiced

Instructions:

1. Wash all produce thoroughly.
2. Cut the cucumber and apple into slices.
3. Add the spinach, cucumber, apple, and lemon juice to a juicer.
4. Process until smooth.
5. Serve immediately over ice.

This refreshing and tangy juice contains nutrients and antioxidants from spinach, cucumber, apple, and lemon. The spinach provides a good dose of vitamin K, while the cucumber is rich in vitamin C and silica. The apple adds natural sweetness and fiber, and the lemon adds a zesty kick of vitamin C and citric acid. This Green Lemonade is a perfect way to energize and nourish your body while fighting cancer.

- **Spicy Green: kale, celery, green apple, jalapeño, lime**

Here's the recipe for Spicy Green:

Ingredients:

- 2 cups of kale
- 2 celery stalks
- 1 green apple
- 1 jalapeño, seeds removed
- 1 lime, juiced

Instructions:

1. Wash all ingredients thoroughly.
2. Cut the kale leaves off the stem and discard the stem.
3. Cut the celery stalks into small pieces.
4. Cut the green apple into quarters and remove the core.
5. Cut the jalapeño in half, remove the seeds, and cut into small pieces.
6. Juice all the ingredients, including the lime, in a juicer.

7. Pour the juice into a glass and stir well.
8. Serve immediately and enjoy the spicy kick!

This recipe is delicious and packed with cancer-fighting nutrients like vitamin C, beta-carotene, and sulforaphane. The spicy kick from the jalapeño adds a unique flavor. Also, it helps boost metabolism and reduce inflammation in the body. It's the perfect juice to start your day or to give you an energy boost during the day.

- **Berry Beet: beets, raspberries, blueberries, apples, lemon**

Ingredients:

- 1 large beet, peeled and chopped
- 1 cup raspberries
- 1 cup blueberries
- 1 green apple, cored and chopped
- 1 lemon, juiced

Instructions:

1. Wash and prep all ingredients.

2. To your juicer, add the chopped beet, then the raspberries, blueberries, green apples, and lemon juice.
3. Run everything through the juicer and mix well.
4. Serve immediately over ice.

Enjoy this delicious and nutrient-rich juice, filled with antioxidants and anti-inflammatory properties to help boost your immune system and fight cancer.

- **Carrot Pineapple: carrots, pineapple, ginger, and lemon**

Ingredients:

- 4 medium-sized carrots
- 1/4 pineapple
- 1/2 inch ginger
- 1/2 lemon

Instructions:

1. Wash and chop the carrots, pineapple, and ginger into small pieces.
2. Add the chopped ingredients into a juicer and juice.
3. Squeeze in the juice from half a lemon.
4. Stir the juice and pour it into a glass.

5. Serve and enjoy the refreshing taste of Carrot Pineapple juice.

- **Turmeric Tonic: turmeric, ginger, lemon, honey**

Here's the recipe for the Turmeric Tonic:

Ingredients:

- 1-inch fresh turmeric root, peeled and chopped
- 1-inch fresh ginger root, peeled and chopped
- 1 lemon, juiced
- 1 tablespoon honey
- 2 cups of water

Instructions:

1. In a blender, combine the chopped turmeric and ginger with 2 cups of water. Blend until smooth.
2. Strain the mixture through a fine-mesh strainer, into a bowl or pitcher.
3. Add the lemon juice and honey, and stir well.
4. Serve immediately over ice or store in the fridge for up to 3 days.

This tonic is packed with anti-inflammatory and immune-boosting properties from turmeric and ginger. The lemon juice adds a dose of vitamin C, while the honey adds a touch of sweetness. Enjoy this refreshing and health-promoting drink as a part of your cancer treatment plan.

- **Melon Medley: honeydew, cantaloupe, cucumber, mint**

Ingredients:

- 1 cup honeydew, cubed
- 1 cup cantaloupe, cubed
- 1 small cucumber, chopped
- 1 tablespoon of fresh mint leaves
- 1 cup of ice

Directions:

1. Combine the honeydew, cantaloupe, cucumber, and mint leaves in a blender.
2. Add ice and blend until smooth.
3. Pour into a glass and serve immediately.

This refreshing juice is loaded with vitamins, minerals, and antioxidants that can help boost your immune system and fight against cancer.

The honeydew and cantaloupe provide a good source of vitamin C, while the cucumber and mint leaves help to soothe the digestive system. Enjoy this Melon Medley juice as a healthy and delicious way to stay hydrated and nourished.

- **Orange Carrot Ginger: oranges, carrots, ginger, lemon**

Orange Carrot Ginger Recipe:

Ingredients:

- 4 medium-sized carrots, chopped
- 2 oranges, peeled and segmented
- 1 small piece of ginger, peeled and chopped
- 1/2 lemon, juiced

Instructions:

1. Wash and prepare the carrots, oranges, and ginger.
2. Feed the carrots, oranges, and ginger through a juicer.
3. Squeeze the lemon juice into the juice and stir well.
4. Serve the juice over ice, and enjoy!

This juice recipe is packed with vitamin C, which can help boost the immune system and protect against cancer. Carrots are a great source of beta-carotene, which may help reduce the risk of developing certain types of cancer.

Ginger has anti-inflammatory properties that help reduce inflammation in the body, which is often associated with cancer. Combining sweet oranges and spicy ginger makes a delicious and refreshing juice, perfect for a hot summer day.

Royal Nectar: A mix of golden kiwi, pineapple, and turmeric for a sweet, anti-inflammatory drink that supports immune function and fights cancer.

Ingredients:

- 2 golden kiwis
- 1 cup of fresh pineapple chunks
- 1 teaspoon of ground turmeric
- 1 cup of water

Instructions:

1. Peel the golden kiwis and cut them into chunks.
2. Cut the fresh pineapple into small pieces.
3. Add the golden kiwi and pineapple pieces to a juicer.
4. Add the ground turmeric to the juicer.
5. Turn the juicer on and let it run until all the ingredients are well blended and juiced.
6. Pour the juice into a glass and serve immediately.

Royal Nectar is a refreshing and delicious juice packed with anti-inflammatory compounds and immune-boosting properties. Vitamin C, which is necessary for the immune system and general health, is abundant in golden kiwis. Bromelain is an enzyme found in pineapple that aids in digestion and reduces inflammation. Turmeric is a powerful anti-inflammatory spice that has been shown to have cancer-fighting properties. This juice is a great way to start your day and support your body's natural defenses against cancer.

- **Carrot Cucumber Ginger: carrots, cucumber, ginger, lemon**

Carrot Cucumber Ginger Juice Recipe:

Ingredients:

- 4 large carrots, peeled and chopped
- 1 large cucumber, peeled and chopped
- 1-inch piece of ginger, peeled
- 1 lemon, juiced

Instructions:

1. Wash all produce thoroughly.
2. Peel the carrots and cucumber, and chop them into smaller pieces.
3. Peel the ginger and cut it into smaller pieces.
4. Juice all the ingredients together in a juicer.
5. Squeeze the lemon into the juice and stir.
6. Pour the juice into a glass and enjoy immediately.

This juice is packed with nutrients from carrots, cucumber, and ginger. The lemon adds a nice, tangy flavor and boosts the vitamin C content. This juice is great for aiding digestion and reducing inflammation in the body. It's also a refreshing and hydrating drink to enjoy any time of the day.

- **Green Tea Infusion: green tea, spinach, cucumber, honey**

Ingredients:

- 2 green tea bags
- 1 cup of spinach leaves
- 1 medium cucumber, peeled and chopped
- 1 tablespoon honey
- 1 cup of water

Instructions:

1. Bring water to a boil in a small saucepan.
2. Remove from heat and add green tea bags. Steep for 3-4 minutes.
3. Remove the tea bags and allow the tea to cool to room temperature.
4. In a blender, combine spinach, cucumber, honey, and cooled green tea.
5. Blend until smooth.
6. Serve chilled, and enjoy!

- **Mango Tango: mango, orange, apple, ginger**

Ingredients:

- 2 ripe mangoes, peeled and chopped
- 1 medium-sized apple, cored and chopped
- 1 medium-sized orange, peeled and separated into segments
- 1/2 inch fresh ginger, peeled
- 1 cup of water
- Ice cubes (optional)

Instructions:

1. Wash and chop the mangoes, apples, and oranges into small pieces.
2. Peel the ginger and chop it finely.
3. Add all the chopped fruits and ginger to a juicer or blender.
4. Pour in 1 cup of water and blend everything until smooth.
5. You can strain the juice through a sieve if you prefer a smoother texture.
6. If desired, add ice cubes to chill the juice and serve immediately.

Enjoy your refreshing and nutritious Mango Tango juice!

- **Spicy Pineapple: pineapple, ginger, jalapeño, lemon**

Ingredients:

- 1 pineapple, peeled and chopped
- 1-inch piece of fresh ginger, peeled
- 1 jalapeño pepper, seeded
- 1 lemon, juiced

Instructions:

1. Run the pineapple, ginger, and jalapeño through a juicer.
2. Stir in the lemon juice.
3. Serve over ice.

Note: Adjust the amount of jalapeño based on your preference for spiciness. If you prefer it less spicy, you can remove the seeds or use half of the jalapeño.

- **Red Recovery: beets, carrots, apple, lemon, ginger**

Ingredients:

- 1 medium beet, peeled and chopped

- 2 medium carrots, peeled and chopped
- 1 medium apple, cored and chopped
- 1-inch piece of fresh ginger, peeled
- 1/2 lemon, juiced

Directions:

1. Wash and prepare all ingredients.
2. Add beets, carrots, apples, and ginger to the juicer and juice.
3. Add lemon juice to the mixture and stir.
4. Pour into a glass and enjoy immediately.

Benefits:

This juice is packed with nutrients and antioxidants, making it a great addition to a cancer patient's diet. The beets contain a lot of betalains, which have anti-inflammatory properties and might fend off some cancers. Beta-carotene, abundant in carrots, can strengthen the immune system and lower cancer risk. Due to their high fiber content, apples help digestion and gut health. Ginger has antioxidant and anti-inflammatory qualities, which may help reduce nausea—a frequent side effect of cancer treatments. The vitamin C boost from lemon juice supports the immune system and reduces inflammation.

- **Cucumber Limeade: cucumber, lime, honey**

Here's the recipe for Cucumber Limeade:

Ingredients:

- 2 cucumbers, peeled and chopped
- 3 limes, juiced
- 1/4 cup honey
- 4 cups of water
- Ice

Instructions:

1. In a blender, blend the chopped cucumbers until smooth.
2. Strain the cucumber juice through a fine-mesh sieve into a pitcher.
3. Add the lime juice and honey to the pitcher, and stir well.
4. Add the water and stir again.
5. Chill the limeade in the refrigerator for at least an hour.
6. Serve over ice.

This refreshing juice is perfect for a hot summer day. Cucumbers are hydrating and help to flush toxins out of the body. At the same time, lime is a great source of vitamin C and antioxidants. The honey adds a touch of sweetness, and the water dilutes the juice to create a refreshing, thirst-quenching beverage. Enjoy!

- **Tropical Turmeric: pineapple, mango, turmeric, ginger**

Ingredients:

- 1 cup fresh pineapple chunks
- 1 cup fresh mango chunks
- 1 tsp turmeric powder
- 1-inch piece of fresh ginger, peeled and chopped
- 1 cup water
- 1 tbsp honey (optional)

Instructions:

1. Add the pineapple, mango, turmeric, and ginger to a juicer or blender and blend until smooth.
2. Pour the mixture into a glass.
3. Add water to the mixture to thin it out to your desired consistency.

4. Stir in honey if desired.

5. Serve immediately and enjoy.

Benefits:

This juice is a delicious way to get your daily dose of turmeric, which is a powerful anti-inflammatory agent that may help to prevent cancer growth and reduce inflammation in the body. The addition of fresh pineapple and mango provides natural sweetness and a boost of vitamin C, while ginger adds a spicy kick and helps to settle the stomach. Enjoy this refreshing tropical juice as a healthy and tasty way to support your body's overall health and well-being.

- **Carrot Apple Ginger: carrots, apple, ginger, lemon**

Carrot Apple Ginger is a refreshing and healthy juice recipe that is packed with nutrients and antioxidants. This delicious juice is perfect for a quick breakfast or mid-day snack to keep you energized and focused.

Ingredients:

- 4 large carrots

- 2 apples
- 1 inch of ginger
- 1/2 lemon (optional)

Instructions:

1. Wash all the ingredients thoroughly.
2. Cut the carrots and apples into small pieces fit into your juicer.
3. Ginger should be peeled and chopped into smaller pieces.
4. Juice all the ingredients in a juicer.
5. Stir the juice well.
6. Add lemon juice (optional) and serve over ice.

This juice is not only delicious but also highly nutritious. Carrots are loaded with beta-carotene, which is an antioxidant that is beneficial for your eyesight and skin. Ginger is well-known for its anti-inflammatory properties, and apples are a fantastic source of fiber and vitamins. The lemon juice is optional but adds a nice tangy flavor to the juice and is a great source of vitamin C.

This carrot, apple, and ginger juice is a wonderful addition to any diet. It helps strengthen your immune system, enhances digestion, and energizes you all day.

- **Berry Boost: blueberries, strawberries, raspberries, almond milk**

Ingredients:

- 1 cup of blueberries
- 1 cup of strawberries
- 1 cup of raspberries
- 1 cup of almond milk
- 1 teaspoon of honey (optional)

Instructions:

1. Wash all the berries and blend them in a juicer or blender until smooth.
2. Add almond milk and blend again until smooth.
3. Taste and add honey if desired.
4. Enjoy your delicious Berry Boost juice after pouring it into a glass!

- **Green Machine 2.0: kale, cucumber, celery, green apple, lemon, parsley**

Green Machine 2.0 is a juice that packs a serious nutritional punch. This delicious blend is made with kale, cucumber, celery, green apple, lemon, and parsley. This recipe is great for enhancing your general well-being because each ingredient has special health benefits.

The cruciferous vegetable kale is an abundant source of vitamins and minerals, such as iron, vitamin C, and vitamin K. It has anti-inflammatory and antioxidant substances that help lower the risk of developing certain cancers. Because they are high in water and fiber and low in calories, cucumbers are a great option for digestion and weight loss. They are also rich in antioxidants and help reduce inflammation in the body.

Celery is another low-calorie vegetable that is packed with nutrients. It is high in fiber and may help lower cholesterol levels and reduce inflammation. Because they lower the risk of heart disease, green apples, which are highly antioxidants, help improve heart health. Additionally, they contain pectin, a fiber that aids in fostering feelings of fullness.

The citrus fruit lemon contains a lot of antioxidants and vitamin C. It may help improve digestion and boost the immune system.

Vitamins A, C, and K, as well as antioxidants, are abundant in the herb parsley. It may also have anti-inflammatory properties and may help improve kidney function.

Ingredients:

- 2 cups kale leaves, chopped
- 1 medium cucumber, chopped
- 2 stalks of celery, chopped
- 1 green apple, chopped
- 1 lemon, juiced
- 1/4 cup fresh parsley leaves

Instructions:

1. Wash all produce thoroughly.
2. Chop the kale, cucumber, celery, and green apple into small pieces.
3. Add the chopped ingredients to a juicer and juice them.
4. Pour the juice into a glass.
5. Juice the lemon, then pour it into your glass.
6. Finely chop the fresh parsley leaves and sprinkle them over the juice.
7. Stir the juice and parsley together.
8. Enjoy your Green Machine 2.0 juice!

Together, these ingredients create a juice that is both delicious and nutritious. Green Machine 2.0 is a great way to start your day; it provides a burst of energy and helps keep you full and satisfied. Try this recipe out and see how your health and well-being will improve.

- **Ginger Lemon Blast: ginger, lemon, and honey**

Ginger Lemon Blast is a delicious, refreshing juice with a powerful nutritional punch. This simple yet potent juice is made with only three ingredients: ginger, lemon, and honey. Compared to lemon, which is rich in vitamin C and antioxidants, ginger is well known for its anti-inflammatory and immune-boosting qualities. In addition to having natural sweetness and antibacterial and anti-inflammatory properties, honey is a great addition.

To make Ginger Lemon Blast:
1. Peel and chop a small piece of fresh ginger root.
2. To a glass, add the ginger and squeeze the juice of one lemon.
3. Mix well, then add a teaspoon of honey, stirring until it dissolves. You can make

the juice as sweet or as potent as you like by varying the amounts of honey and ginger.

This juice is great for a morning pick-me-up or an energy boost in the afternoon. Due to its immune-boosting qualities, it's also fantastic at warding off colds and the flu. So the next time you need a quick and nutritious juice, try Ginger Lemon Blast and experience it's revitalizing and reviving effects.

- **Apple Cider Vinegar Tonic: apple cider vinegar, lemon, honey, cinnamon**

Since ancient times, people have used apple cider vinegar for its plethora of health advantages, which include enhancing digestion, lowering inflammation, and promoting weight loss. When combined with other powerful ingredients, such as lemon, honey, and cinnamon, it can create a potent tonic to help fight illness and promote overall health.

Recipe for an Apple Cider Vinegar Tonic:

Ingredients:

- 1 tablespoon apple cider vinegar

- 1 tablespoon fresh lemon juice
- 1 teaspoon honey
- 1/4 teaspoon cinnamon
- 1 cup of water

Instructions:

1. Mix the apple cider vinegar, lemon juice, honey, and cinnamon in a glass.
2. Add water and stir well.
3. Drink it immediately or put it in the refrigerator for up to 24 hours.

Use this tonic daily for the best results as a great way to start your day. Combining apple cider vinegar, lemon, honey, and cinnamon creates a refreshing and delicious drink that can help improve your health and well-being.

- **Pineapple Cucumber Mint: pineapple, cucumber, mint, and lemon**

Pineapple Cucumber Mint is a refreshing and delicious juice recipe that is perfect for a hot summer day. It is packed with vitamins, minerals, and antioxidants that help to boost your immune system and improve your overall health. Cucumber is a great source of vitamin K, which aids in blood clotting and bone health, whereas pineapple is a great source of vitamin C, which is necessary for the synthesis of collagen.

Mint is another excellent addition because it is a natural stimulant that can aid in nausea relief and digestive system calming. Finally, lemon adds a tart and tangy flavor while providing vitamin C and antioxidants.

You will need 1 cup of chopped pineapple, 1 cucumber, 10-12 fresh mint leaves, and 1 lemon to make this recipe. Begin by peeling the cucumber and cutting it into chunks. Then, add the cucumber, pineapple, and mint leaves to a juicer and process until smooth. Lemon juice should be squeezed and added to the juice mixture. Stir in some ice and enjoy your delicious and nutritious Pineapple Cucumber Mint juice!

- **Carrot Orange Pineapple: carrots, orange, pineapple, ginger**

Carrot Orange Pineapple Juice Recipe:

Ingredients:

- 4 large carrots, peeled and chopped
- 1 orange, peeled and segmented
- 1 cup fresh pineapple, chopped
- Peeled and grated ginger, 1 inch long.
- 1/2 cup of water

Instructions:

1. Add the chopped carrots, orange segments, and pineapple to a juicer.
2. Add the grated ginger and water to the juicer.
3. Turn on the juicer and juice all the ingredients together.
4. Once all the juice is extracted, give it a good stir.
5. Enjoy the juice by pouring it into a glass.

The juice contains minerals and vitamins from carrots, oranges, and pineapple. At the same time, the ginger adds a spicy kick and aids digestion. It's perfect for starting your day on a healthy note or as an afternoon pick-me-up.

- **Ginger Peach: peaches, ginger, lemon**

Ginger Peach is a flavorful and reviving juice combining the sweetness of peaches with the zing of ginger and the tang of lemon. This juice is a great way to start the day because it is full of vitamins and antioxidants, or you can enjoy it as a healthy snack.
To make Ginger Peach juice, you will need the following:

- 3 ripe peaches, pitted and sliced
- 1-inch piece of fresh peeled and chopped ginger
- 1 lemon, juiced

Instructions:

1. Wash and prepare all the ingredients.
2. In a juicer, add the sliced peaches and chopped ginger.
3. Juice the peaches and ginger according to your juicer's instructions.
4. Add the lemon juice to the juicer and stir well.

5. Enjoy the juice after pouring it into a glass.

Ginger Peach juice is a fantastic source of vitamin C, which can help your body fight off infections and strengthen your immune system. Additionally anti-inflammatory, ginger can help with nausea relief and digestive problems. Vitamin A, which supports healthy vision and skin, dietary fiber, and potassium are all present in peaches in good amounts. Any time of day is a good time to drink this tasty and healthy juice.

- **Beet Berry Basil: beets, raspberries, blueberries, basil, and lemon**

Ingredients:

- 1 small beet, peeled and chopped
- 1/2 cup raspberries
- 1/2 cup blueberries
- 2-3 fresh basil leaves
- 1/2 lemon, juiced
- 1 cup of water or coconut water

Instructions:

1. Juice until smooth after adding all ingredients to a juicer.
2. Add more water or coconut water until the desired consistency is reached if the juice is too thick.
3. Serve immediately and enjoy!

- **Green Detox: kale, spinach, cucumber, celery, green apple, lemon**

A Green Detox smoothie is a nutrient-packed drink to help you feel refreshed and rejuvenated. Here's a recipe for you to try:

Ingredients:

- 1 cup of kale
- 1 cup of spinach
- 1/2 cucumber
- 2 celery stalks
- 1 green apple
- 1/2 lemon, juiced
- 1 cup water

Instructions:

1. Wash and chop all ingredients.
2. Add them to a juicer with 1 cup of water.
3. Juice until smooth and creamy.

4. If needed, add more water to achieve the desired consistency.
5. Enjoy your delicious and nutritious Green Detox smoothie!

* **Spicy Apple: apples, jalapeño, lime, honey**

Ingredients:

* 2 medium apples, cored and chopped
* 1 small jalapeño, seeded and chopped
* 1 lime, juiced
* 1 tablespoon honey
* 1/2 cup water
* 1 cup of ice cubes

1. **Apples should be washed, cored, and cut into small pieces.**
2. Cut the jalapeno pepper into small pieces and remove the seeds (optional).
3. Juice the apples and jalapenos in a juicer.
4. Squeeze the lime juice into the juice and mix well.
5. Add honey to taste and stir until it dissolves.
6. Pour the juice into a glass and enjoy!

Note: Depending on how hot you want the juice to be, change the amount of jalapeno pepper to your preference. Include some ice cubes in the juice for refreshing summer juice.

- **Watermelon Lime Mint: watermelon, lime, mint.**

A Watermelon Lime Mint is a refreshing and hydrating drink perfect for hot summer days. Here's how to make it:

Ingredients:

- 24 cups of chopped watermelon
- 1 lime, juiced
- A handful of fresh mint leaves
- Ice cubes

Equipment:

- Juicer
- Pitcher
- Stirring spoon

Instructions:

1. Wash and chop the watermelon into small pieces.
2. Juice the watermelon using a juicer.
3. The lime should be juiced and added to the watermelon juice.
4. Wash the mint leaves and chop them finely. Add the mint leaves to the juice.
5. Stir the juice well to combine all the ingredients.
6. Add ice cubes to the juice and stir again.
7. Juice should be poured into a pitcher and served right away.

Enjoy your refreshing Watermelon Lime Mint juice!

- **Carrot Ginger Lime: carrots, ginger, lime**

Carrot Ginger Lime juice is a delicious and refreshing drink perfect for a hot summer day. This juice is made with fresh carrots, ginger, and lime, which give it a zesty and tangy flavor.

To make this juice, peel and chop the carrots and ginger into small pieces. Then, juice the carrots and ginger using a juicer or blender. Once the juice is ready, add the juice of one lime and stir well.

If you want to sweeten the juice even more, add a little honey or maple syrup. Serve the carrot ginger, and lime juice over ice and top with a lime slice or fresh mint sprig for decoration. Enjoy!

- **Golden Elixir: A blend of turmeric, ginger, carrot, and orange to boost immunity and reduce inflammation.**

Golden Elixir is a nutrient-dense smoothie that combines the benefits of turmeric, ginger, carrot, and orange to support a healthy immune system and reduce inflammation. While carrots are high in beta-carotene, a potent antioxidant, turmeric, ginger, and both are recognized for their anti-inflammatory properties. Oranges contain a lot of vitamin C, which improves immunity and lowers the chance of infection. These ingredients work together to produce a delicious and revitalizing juice that tastes great and is healthy.

Ingredients:
- 1 medium-sized turmeric root
- 1 small piece of ginger root
- 4 medium-sized carrots
- 2 oranges

Instructions:

1. Peel the turmeric and ginger roots and chop them into small pieces.
2. Carrots should be washed and cut into small pieces.
3. Peel the oranges and separate the segments.
4. Add the turmeric, ginger, carrots, and oranges to a juicer.
5. Juice all the ingredients until well blended.
6. In a glass, pour the juice and give it a good stir.

Drink immediately for the best taste and maximum health benefits.

- **Berry Blast: A mix of strawberries, blueberries, raspberries, and spinach for a powerful antioxidant boost.**

The combination of these berries provides a great source of vitamins and antioxidants, and spinach adds some extra nutritional value. Here's a possible recipe:

Ingredients:

- 1 cup strawberries
- 1 cup of blueberries
- 1 cup raspberries
- 2 cups of fresh spinach
- 1 cup of water or almond milk
- 1-2 tablespoons honey (optional)

Instructions:

1. Rinse all fruits and spinach and pat dry.
2. Add all ingredients to a blender and blend until smooth.
3. Taste and add honey if desired for extra sweetness.
4. Pour into a glass and enjoy your delicious and healthy Berry Blast!

Sunset Serenade: A delicious blend of grapefruit, orange, and carrot, rich in vitamin C and beta-carotene.

Sunset Serenade is a refreshing and nutritious juice perfect for any time of day. This blend will surely please your taste buds with a beautiful orange hue and a sweet and tangy flavor.

Grapefruit is packed with vitamin C, which helps to support the immune system and can reduce inflammation. It also contains antioxidants to help protect against cellular damage and may reduce the risk of chronic diseases.

Oranges are another excellent vitamin C source and contain fiber, which helps support digestion and promote feelings of fullness.

Carrots are rich in beta-carotene, converted into vitamin A in the body. This nutrient is essential for healthy vision and can also help support the immune system.

Ingredients:

- 1 grapefruit
- 2 oranges
- 2 carrots

Instructions:

1. Peel the grapefruit and oranges and remove any seeds.
2. Wash the carrots and cut off the ends.

3. Cut the grapefruit, oranges, and carrots into small pieces that will fit into your juicer.
4. Feed the fruit and vegetables through your juicer.
5. Stir the juice well and serve immediately.

Enjoy your delicious Sunset Serenade juice, packed with vitamins and antioxidants to support your health and well-being!

- **Green Monster: A mix of kale, cucumber, celery, and green apple for a nutrient-dense and alkalizing juice.**

Green Monster: Packed with nutrients and a natural alkalizer, this juice blends kale, cucumber, celery, and green apple. Combining these ingredients provides a refreshing and energizing drink that is perfect for a healthy start to your day or as a post-workout drink. Enjoy the benefits of greens and the hydrating effects of cucumber and apple in one tasty juice.

Here's how you can prepare Green Monster juice:

Ingredients:

- 1 bunch of kale

- 1 cucumber
- 3 stalks of celery
- 1 green apple

Instructions:

1. Wash all ingredients thoroughly.
2. Remove the stem from the kale leaves.
3. Cut the cucumber, celery, and green apple into pieces that fit your juicer.
4. Add the ingredients to your juicer and process.
5. Serve the juice immediately for the best flavor and nutrient content.

Note: If you don't have a juicer, you can use a blender to make a smoothie instead. Simply add a small amount of water or other liquid to help blend the ingredients together.

- **Sweet & Spicy: A blend of sweet potato, carrot, ginger, and cinnamon to regulate blood sugar levels and reduce inflammation.**

To prepare Sweet & Spicy juice, follow these simple steps:

1. Wash and chop 1 medium-sized sweet potato and 2-3 medium-sized carrots into small pieces.
2. Peel and chop a 1-inch piece of fresh ginger.
3. Add the chopped sweet potato, carrots, and ginger into a juicer.
4. Run the juicer until all the ingredients are blended and juiced.
5. Pour the juice into a glass.
6. Sprinkle a pinch of cinnamon on top and stir well.
7. Enjoy the Sweet & Spicy juice immediately for maximum freshness and nutritional benefits.

- **Lemon-Lime Refresher: A mix of lemon, lime, cucumber, and mint to aid digestion and support liver function.**

To make Lemon-Lime Refresher, start by juicing 1 lemon and 1 lime. Add the juice to a blender with 1 sliced cucumber and a handful of fresh mint leaves. Blend until smooth, then strain the mixture through a fine mesh strainer or cheesecloth. Serve over ice and enjoy it as a refreshing and healthful drink.

- **Purple Reign: A blend of beets, blueberries, and kale, rich in antioxidants and anti-inflammatory compounds**

Purple Reign is a delicious and nutritious juice that combines the goodness of beets, blueberries, and kale. This juice is packed with antioxidants and anti-inflammatory compounds, making it an excellent choice for promoting overall health and well-being.

Ingredients:

- 1 medium-sized beet
- 1 cup of blueberries
- 2-3 kale leaves
- ½ lemon (juiced)
- 1-inch piece of ginger (optional)

Instructions:

1. Wash all the ingredients thoroughly under running water.
2. Cut the beet into small pieces that can fit into your juicer.
3. Remove the stems from the kale leaves and cut them into smaller pieces.

4. Add the beet, blueberries, and kale to your juicer.
5. Extract the juice and collect it in a glass.
6. Add the freshly squeezed lemon juice and stir well.
7. If you prefer a bit of spice, you can also add a 1-inch piece of ginger to the juicer.

Tips:

- It's important to use fresh ingredients when making this juice to get the maximum nutritional benefit.
- You can adjust the amount of each ingredient to suit your taste preferences.
- If you don't have a juicer, you can use a blender to make a smoothie instead. Simply blend all the ingredients together and strain out any pulp.
- You can also add some ice cubes to your juice to make it more refreshing on hot days.

Overall, Purple Reign is a delicious and healthy juice that you can enjoy at any time of the day. With its powerful antioxidant and anti-inflammatory properties, this juice can help support your immune system and promote overall wellness.

- **Pineapple Paradise: A pineapple, ginger, and turmeric mix to aid digestion and reduce inflammation.**

Pineapple Paradise is a delicious juice that combines the sweet and tangy flavor of pineapple with the spicy kick of ginger and the earthy notes of turmeric. This juice is not only tasty but also packed with health benefits. Pineapple contains an enzyme called bromelain, which can help improve digestion and reduce inflammation. Ginger is a natural anti-inflammatory and can also aid in digestion. Turmeric is known for its anti-inflammatory and antioxidant properties, which can help protect against various chronic diseases.

Here's how to make Pineapple Paradise:

Ingredients:

- 1 cup of fresh pineapple chunks
- 1 inch of fresh ginger root, peeled and chopped
- 1/2 teaspoon of ground turmeric

- 1/2 cup of water

Instructions:

1. Wash the pineapple and cut it into chunks.
2. Peel and chop the ginger root.
3. Add the pineapple, ginger, turmeric, and water to a blender or juicer.
4. Blend or juice the ingredients until smooth.
5. If using a blender, strain the juice through a fine mesh sieve to remove any solids.
6. Serve the Pineapple Paradise juice immediately, garnished with a slice of pineapple or a sprig of fresh mint if desired.

Note: You can adjust the amount of water to your desired consistency. If you prefer a thinner juice, add more water. If you prefer a thicker juice, reduce the amount of water. Additionally, you can add a teaspoon of honey or maple syrup to sweeten the juice, but remember that the pineapple is already naturally sweet.

- **Carrot Cake Delight: A blend of carrot, apple, cinnamon, and nutmeg for a tasty and nutritious treat.**

Carrot Cake Delight is a delicious and healthy juice that tastes like a classic dessert while providing numerous health benefits. The juice is a blend of carrot, apple, cinnamon, and nutmeg, all nutrient-dense ingredients that contribute to its unique flavor and health-promoting properties.

To make Carrot Cake Delight, you will need a juicer, a cutting board, and a sharp knife. Here's how to prepare it:

Ingredients:

- 4 medium-sized carrots, peeled and chopped
- 2 medium-sized apples, cored and chopped
- 1/2 teaspoon cinnamon
- 1/4 teaspoon nutmeg

Instructions:

1. Wash the carrots and apples thoroughly under running water.
2. Peel the carrots and chop them into small pieces.
3. Core the apples and chop them into small pieces.
4. Add the chopped carrots and apples to the juicer.
5. Juice the carrots and apples according to the manufacturer's instructions.
6. Pour the juice into a glass.
7. Add the cinnamon and nutmeg to the juice and stir well.
8. Serve and enjoy!

Carrots are an excellent vitamin A source, essential for maintaining healthy vision, skin, and immune function. They are also rich in fiber, potassium, and antioxidants, which help to lower cholesterol levels and reduce the risk of chronic diseases.

Apples are another nutritious ingredient in this juice. They are a good source of fiber, vitamin C, and antioxidants. Apples have been shown to lower the risk of heart disease, stroke, and cancer.

Cinnamon and nutmeg add warmth and flavor to the juice while providing health benefits. Cinnamon has been shown to lower blood sugar levels, improve insulin sensitivity, and reduce inflammation. Nutmeg is also anti-inflammatory and used in traditional medicine to treat digestive issues and insomnia.

Overall, Carrot Cake Delight is a tasty and nutritious juice that is easy to prepare and packed with health-promoting ingredients. It can be enjoyed as a healthy snack or dessert, satisfying your sweet tooth without compromising your health goals.

- **Sunshine in a Glass: A mix of orange, grapefruit, and lemon to boost immunity and provide a dose of vitamin C**

Sunshine in a Glass is a refreshing and immune-boosting juice that combines the bright and citrusy flavors of orange, grapefruit, and lemon. Here's how you can make it at home:

Ingredients:

- 2 oranges, peeled
- 1 grapefruit, peeled

- 1 lemon, peeled
- Ice cubes (optional)

Instructions:

1. Begin by washing and preparing the fruit. Remove the peel and pith from the oranges, grapefruit, and lemon, and discard.
2. Cut the oranges, grapefruit, and lemon into small pieces that can fit into your juicer.
3. Juice the fruit using a juicer. If you don't have a juicer, you can use a blender to blend the fruit with some water, then strain the juice through a fine-mesh sieve or cheesecloth.
4. If you prefer your juice cold, you can add a few ice cubes to the glass before pouring the juice.

Variations:

- For an even sweeter juice, add a small amount of honey or agave nectar.
- For a spicier kick, add a small piece of ginger to the mix.

- If you don't have all the fruits on hand, you can use any combination of orange, grapefruit, and lemon that you prefer.

Sunshine in a Glass is a delicious and refreshing way to start your day or to give your immune system a boost when you're feeling under the weather.

- **Radiant Recovery: A blend of kale, cucumber, celery, green apple, lemon, ginger, and turmeric for a powerful antioxidant and anti-inflammatory boost.**

Radiant Recovery is a nutrient-dense juice that combines the goodness of kale, cucumber, celery, green apple, lemon, ginger, and turmeric to create a powerful anti-inflammatory and antioxidant boost that can help improve overall health and well-being.

To prepare this juice, you will need:

- 1 cup of kale leaves, washed and chopped
- 1 small cucumber, chopped
- 2 stalks of celery, chopped
- 1 green apple, cored and chopped
- 1 lemon, juiced

- 1 inch of fresh ginger, peeled and chopped
- 1 teaspoon of ground turmeric
- 1 cup of water

Instructions:

1. Add the kale, cucumber, celery, and green apple to a juicer and extract the juice.
2. Pour the juice into a blender.
3. Add the lemon juice, ginger, turmeric, and water to the blender.
4. Blend on high speed until smooth.
5. Serve immediately.

This juice contains vitamins, minerals, and antioxidants that can help reduce inflammation, boost immunity, and support overall health. Kale, cucumber, and celery are rich in antioxidants and anti-inflammatory compounds. At the same time, the green apple adds a touch of sweetness and additional nutrients like vitamin C and fiber. The lemon juice adds a refreshing tang and a boost of vitamin C. At the same time, ginger and turmeric provide powerful anti-inflammatory benefits.

Enjoy Radiant Recovery as a delicious and nutritious way to start your day or as a mid-day pick-me-up to keep you energized and focused.

- **Immune Elixir: A mix of grapefruit, orange, lemon, and ginger to support immune function and reduce inflammation.**

Immune Elixir is a refreshing and powerful juice blend that can help boost your immune system and reduce inflammation. This juice recipe is packed with vitamin C and antioxidants, making it an excellent choice for anyone looking to stay healthy and support their immune system.

Here is how to make this delicious and nutritious Immune Elixir:

Ingredients:

- 1 grapefruit
- 1 orange
- 1 lemon
- 1-inch piece of fresh ginger

Instructions:

1. Peel the grapefruit, orange, and lemon and remove any seeds.
2. Cut the fruits into pieces small enough to fit into your juicer.
3. Peel the ginger and cut it into small pieces.
4. Add all the ingredients to your juicer and process until smooth.
5. Serve immediately and enjoy the refreshing and immune-boosting benefits of this delicious juice.

This juice recipe is a great way to start your day or to enjoy it as a refreshing snack anytime. It is also a perfect option for anyone looking to support their immune system and reduce inflammation naturally.

- **Pink Power: A blend of beets, strawberries, and watermelon for a high dose of antioxidants and anti-inflammatory compounds**

Pink Power Juice Recipe:

Ingredients:

- 1 medium-sized beetroot, peeled and sliced

- 1 cup strawberries, hulled and sliced
- 2 cups watermelon, cubed
- 1 tablespoon fresh ginger, peeled and grated
- 1 tablespoon honey (optional)
- 1 lemon, juiced

Instructions:

1. Wash all the fruits and vegetables thoroughly.
2. Cut the beetroot, strawberries, and watermelon into small pieces.
3. In a juicer, add the beetroot, strawberries, and watermelon and blend until smooth.
4. Add the grated ginger to the juice and blend again.
5. Taste the juice and add honey to sweeten, if needed.
6. Squeeze lemon juice into the juice mixture and stir well.
7. Pour the juice into a glass and serve immediately.

This Pink Power juice is a delicious and nutritious way to boost your body's immune system and protect against inflammation. The beets provide a rich source of antioxidants and anti-inflammatory compounds. At the same time, the strawberries and watermelon add a sweet and refreshing flavor to the juice. The ginger helps to aid digestion and reduce inflammation. The lemon juice adds a zesty kick of vitamin C. Enjoy this juice as a refreshing and healthy pick-me-up anytime.

- **Turmeric Tonic: A mix of turmeric, ginger, lemon, and honey for a powerful anti-inflammatory and immune-boosting blend.**

Turmeric Tonic is a potent and delicious way to get a healthy dose of anti-inflammatory compounds and immune-boosting nutrients. The key ingredient in this recipe is turmeric, a bright yellow spice that has been used for centuries in traditional medicine for its anti-inflammatory and antioxidant properties.

Ingredients:

- 1-2 inch piece of fresh turmeric root
- 1-2 inch piece of fresh ginger root
- Juice of 1/2 lemon
- 1 teaspoon of honey
- 1 cup of water

Instructions:

1. Peel and chop the turmeric and ginger roots into small pieces.
2. Add the chopped turmeric and ginger to a blender or juicer with the water and blend until smooth.
3. Strain the mixture through a fine mesh strainer or cheesecloth to remove any remaining solids.
4. Mix in the lemon juice and honey until well combined.
5. Serve immediately and enjoy the delicious and nutritious benefits of this Turmeric Tonic.

- **Berry Beet Blast: A combination of beets, raspberries, blueberries, and spinach for a powerful antioxidant boost.**

To make a delicious and nutritious Berry Beet Blast, follow these simple steps:

Ingredients:

- 1 medium beet, peeled and chopped
- 1 cup raspberries
- 1 cup blueberries

- 2 cups fresh spinach
- 1 cup water

Instructions:

1. Add the chopped beet, raspberries, blueberries, and spinach to a blender.
2. Add one cup of water to the blender.
3. Blend the ingredients until the mixture is smooth and well combined.
4. If the mixture is too thick, add a little more water until you reach the desired consistency.
5. Pour the juice into glasses and enjoy immediately.

This juice is a great way to boost your antioxidant intake and support your overall health. The beets add a rich source of dietary nitrates, which can help lower blood pressure and improve exercise performance. Raspberries and blueberries provide an abundance of polyphenols and anthocyanins, which have been shown to have anti-inflammatory and anti-cancer properties. The spinach adds extra vitamins and minerals, including iron and folate. This juice is a great way to start your day on a healthy note or to give your body a midday pick-me-up.

- **Carrot Ginger Sunrise: A mix of carrots, ginger, orange, and lemon for a refreshing and immune-boosting blend.**

Carrot Ginger Sunrise is a delicious and refreshing juice blend that is packed with immune-boosting nutrients.

To prepare the Carrot Ginger Sunrise juice, you will need:

- 4 large carrots, washed and chopped
- 1-inch piece of fresh ginger, peeled and chopped
- 1 orange, peeled and segmented
- 1/2 lemon, peeled and seeded

Instructions:

1. Add the chopped carrots and ginger to a juicer and juice until all the liquid has been extracted.
2. Add the orange segments and lemon to the juicer and juice again.
3. Stir the juice well to combine all the ingredients.

4. Serve the juice immediately over ice for a refreshing drink.

This juice is perfect for a morning pick-me-up. It can help support immune function with its high vitamin C and antioxidant content from oranges and carrots. The ginger also adds a warming and spicy kick, packed with beta-carotene and anti-inflammatory compounds. At the same time, the lemon helps balance out the sweetness of the carrots and oranges.

- **Green Goddess: A blend of kale, spinach, cucumber, celery, green apple, and lemon for a nutrient-dense and alkalizing juice.**

To prepare the Green Goddess juice, follow these steps:

Ingredients:

- 1 cup of kale leaves
- 1 cup of spinach leaves
- 1 medium-sized cucumber, peeled and sliced
- 2-3 celery stalks, chopped
- 1 green apple, cored and sliced

- Juice of 1 lemon

Instructions:

1. Wash all the ingredients properly and chop them into small pieces.
2. Pass the kale, spinach, cucumber, and celery through a juicer.
3. Add the green apple slices and continue to juice until all the ingredients are well blended.
4. Add the lemon juice to the mixture and stir well.
5. Pour the juice into a glass and enjoy!

The Green Goddess juice is packed with vitamins, minerals, and antioxidants, making it an excellent choice for a healthy and refreshing drink. It is an excellent source of chlorophyll, which is known to detoxify the body and support liver function. The lemon juice adds a zesty flavor to the juice while providing vitamin C, which boosts immunity and promotes healthy skin.

- **Orange Blossom: A mix of oranges, carrots, and ginger for a delicious and nutritious blend.**

To prepare Orange Blossom juice, you will need:

Ingredients:

- 2 oranges, peeled and chopped
- 2 medium-sized carrots, peeled and chopped
- 1-inch piece of fresh ginger, peeled and chopped

Instructions:

1. Wash and prepare the ingredients as indicated above.
2. Add the chopped oranges, carrots, and ginger to a juicer.
3. Juice the ingredients until smooth.
4. If desired, strain the juice through a fine-mesh strainer to remove any pulp.
5. Pour the juice into a glass and enjoy immediately.

Note: You can adjust the sweetness of the juice by adding more or less carrots to the mix.

- **Spicy Carrot Ginger: A mix of carrots, ginger, jalapeno, and lemon for a spicy and immune-boosting blend.**

To make Spicy Carrot Ginger juice, you will need:

- 5 medium-sized carrots
- 1-inch piece of ginger
- 1 jalapeno pepper
- 1/2 lemon

Instructions:

1. Wash and chop the carrots into small pieces.
2. Peel and chop the ginger into small pieces.
3. Slice the jalapeno pepper in half and remove the seeds.
4. Juice the carrots, ginger, and jalapeno pepper in a juicer.
5. Squeeze the juice from the lemon into the mix.
6. Stir well and pour into a glass.
7. Add ice if desired and enjoy the spicy and immune-boosting Spicy Carrot Ginger juice!

- **Blueberry Basil Bliss: A combination of blueberries, basil, lemon, and honey for a refreshing and antioxidant-rich blend**

To prepare Blueberry Basil Bliss juice, follow these steps:

Ingredients:

- 1 cup of fresh blueberries
- 2-3 sprigs of fresh basil
- 1/2 lemon, peeled
- 1 teaspoon of honey
- 1/2 cup of water

Instructions:

1. Rinse the blueberries and basil sprigs in water and remove any stems.
2. Peel the lemon and cut it into small pieces.
3. Add the blueberries, basil, lemon, and honey into a blender.
4. Add water to the blender.
5. Blend all the ingredients until smooth.
6. Pour the juice into a glass.

7. Enjoy the refreshing and antioxidant-rich Blueberry Basil Bliss juice.

- **Mango Tango Twist: A blend of mango, orange, pineapple, and coconut water for a delicious and immune-boosting juice.**

To make Mango Tango Twist, you will need:

- 1 large ripe mango, peeled and chopped
- 1 large orange, peeled and segmented
- 1 cup chopped pineapple
- 1 cup coconut water
- Ice cubes

Instructions:

1. Wash and prepare the fruit as needed.
2. Add the mango, orange, and pineapple to a juicer or blender.
3. Blend the fruits until they are smooth.
4. Pour the mixture into a glass.
5. Add coconut water and stir well.
6. Add ice cubes to the glass, if desired.
7. Garnish with a slice of orange or a sprig of mint, and enjoy your delicious and nutritious Mango Tango Twist!

- **Pineapple Cucumber Mint: A mix of pineapple, cucumber, mint, and lemon for a refreshing and antioxidant-rich blend**

Ingredients:

- 1 cup of fresh pineapple chunks
- 1 medium-sized cucumber, chopped
- 1 tablespoon of fresh mint leaves
- Juice of 1 lemon

Instructions:

1. Wash and prepare all the ingredients.
2. Add the pineapple chunks, chopped cucumber, and mint leaves to a juicer or blender.
3. Blend or juice the ingredients until smooth.
4. Add the lemon juice and mix well.
5. Serve the juice over ice and garnish with additional mint leaves, if desired.

Pineapple Cucumber Mint juice is a refreshing and hydrating drink rich in antioxidants and anti-inflammatory compounds. The pineapple and cucumber provide a good source of vitamin C, while the mint and lemon add a burst of flavor. This juice is perfect for hot summer days or as a post-workout drink to rehydrate and replenish the body.

- **Ginger Peach Punch: A blend of peaches, ginger, and lemon for a refreshing and immune-boosting blend**

To prepare Ginger Peach Punch, follow these steps:

Ingredients:

- 2-3 ripe peaches, pitted and chopped
- 1-2 inches of fresh ginger root, peeled and chopped
- Juice of 1 lemon
- 1-2 cups of water
- Honey (optional)

Instructions:

1. Add the chopped peaches and ginger to a blender.
2. Squeeze the lemon juice and add it to the blender.

3. Add 1-2 cups of water and blend until smooth.
4. If the mixture is too thick, add more water until you get the desired consistency.
5. Taste and adjust the sweetness by adding honey, if desired.
6. Serve over ice and enjoy!

- **Acai Berry Blast: A mix of acai berries, blueberries, raspberries, and almond milk for a powerful antioxidant and anti-inflammatory blend**

Ingredients:

- 1 pack of frozen acai berries
- 1/2 cup of blueberries
- 1/2 cup of raspberries
- 1 cup of almond milk
- 1 tablespoon of honey (optional)

Instructions:

1. Run the pack of frozen acai berries under hot water for a few seconds to thaw them out.

2. In a blender, combine the thawed acai berries, blueberries, raspberries, and almond milk.
3. Blend the ingredients until smooth and well combined.
4. Taste the mixture and add honey if desired, blending again until well combined.
5. Pour the juice into glasses and serve immediately.

This Acai Berry Blast is a perfect blend of antioxidants, anti-inflammatory compounds, and healthy fats from almond milk. It is a great way to start your day or to have it as a snack between meals.

- **Grapefruit Ginger Zinger: A combination of grapefruit, ginger, lemon, and honey for a zesty and immune-boosting blend**

To prepare Grapefruit Ginger Zinger juice, you will need the following ingredients:

- 1 grapefruit, peeled and sliced
- 1-inch piece of fresh ginger, peeled and chopped

- 1 lemon, juiced
- 1 tablespoon of honey
- 1 cup of water

Instructions:

1. Add the grapefruit slices, chopped ginger, lemon juice, and honey to a blender.
2. Pour in the water and blend until smooth.
3. Strain the juice through a fine-mesh sieve into a glass.
4. Enjoy immediately for the most health benefits.

This juice contains vitamin C, antioxidants, and anti-inflammatory compounds that can help boost your immune system and fight illness. Ginger and honey also have natural antibacterial and antiviral properties that keep you healthy.

- **Cucumber Lemon Cooler: A cucumber, lemon, and honey mix for a refreshing and immune-boosting blend**

Ingredients:

- 1 cucumber
- 1 lemon

- 1 tablespoon honey
- 1 cup of water

Instructions:

1. Wash the cucumber and lemon thoroughly.
2. Peel the cucumber and cut it into small pieces.
3. Cut the lemon into halves and squeeze the juice into a blender.
4. Add the cucumber pieces, honey, and water to the blender.
5. Blend the ingredients until smooth.
6. Pour the mixture into a glass and add ice cubes if desired.
7. Serve chilled and enjoy your refreshing and immune-boosting Cucumber Lemon Cooler.

- **Kiwi Kale Crush: A blend of kiwi, kale, green apple, and lemon for a nutrient-dense and immune-boosting juice.**

To make Kiwi Kale Crush, you will need the following ingredients:

- 2 kiwis, peeled and sliced

- 1 cup of chopped kale
- 1 green apple, cored and sliced
- 1/2 lemon, juiced

Instructions:

1. Wash and prepare all the ingredients.
2. Add the kiwis, kale, and green apple to a juicer.
3. Juice the ingredients and collect the juice in a glass.
4. Squeeze the lemon juice into the glass and stir to combine.
5. Serve immediately and enjoy your nutrient-dense and immune-boosting Kiwi Kale Crush.

- **Orange Ginger Spice: A mix of oranges, ginger, cinnamon, and honey for a spicy and immune-boosting blend**

Ingredients:

- 3 oranges
- 1-inch piece of fresh ginger
- 1/2 teaspoon ground cinnamon
- 1 tablespoon honey

Instructions:

1. Peel and chop the oranges and ginger.
2. Place the oranges, ginger, and cinnamon in a juicer and juice until smooth.
3. Transfer the juice to a glass.
4. Add the honey and stir until well combined.
5. Serve and enjoy!

This juice is packed with vitamin C from the oranges, and the ginger and cinnamon provide anti-inflammatory and immune-boosting benefits. The honey adds a touch of sweetness and additional health benefits.

- **Strawberry Basil Sipper: A combination of strawberries, basil, and lemon for a refreshing and antioxidant-rich blend**

To prepare a Strawberry Basil Sipper, you will need:

- 1 cup of fresh strawberries
- 1 handful of fresh basil leaves
- 1/2 lemon
- 1 tsp honey (optional)
- 1/2 cup of water

Instructions:

1. Wash and chop the strawberries and basil leaves.
2. Juice the 1/2 lemon and add it to the chopped strawberries and basil in a blender.
3. Add 1 tsp of honey, if desired, and 1/2 cup of water to the blender.
4. Blend all the ingredients until smooth.
5. Strain the mixture through a fine mesh strainer to remove any solids.
6. Serve the juice over ice, garnished with a strawberry and basil leaf, if desired.

Enjoy the refreshing and antioxidant-rich Strawberry Basil Sipper!

- **Lemon Lime Refresher: A mix of lemon, lime, cucumber, and mint to aid digestion and support liver function.**

Lemon Lime Refresher is a simple and refreshing juice that combines the zesty flavors of lemon and lime with the cooling properties of cucumber and mint. This blend is not only delicious, but it also supports digestive health and promotes healthy liver function.

Here's how to make Lemon Lime Refresher:

Ingredients:

- 2 lemons, peeled
- 2 limes, peeled
- 1 cucumber
- 1/2 cup fresh mint leaves
- 1 cup water (optional)

Instructions:

1. Cut the lemons, limes, and cucumber into small pieces that will fit into your juicer.
2. Add the lemon, lime, cucumber, and mint leaves into your juicer and juice until everything is well blended.
3. If the juice is too thick, add 1 cup of water and blend again.
4. Serve the juice immediately over ice.

The Lemon Lime Refresher is perfect for a hot summer day or whenever you want a refreshing and healthy drink. The lemon and lime add a tartness balanced by the cucumber's sweetness, and the mint leaves add a cooling and soothing element. This juice also promotes healthy digestion and liver function, making it a perfect addition to any detox program.

- **Apple Cider Vinegar Tonic: A blend of apple cider vinegar, lemon, honey, and cinnamon for a powerful immune-boosting and anti-inflammatory blend.**

Apple Cider Vinegar Tonic is a popular juice that offers numerous health benefits. It's made from a blend of apple cider vinegar, lemon, honey, and cinnamon, which all have unique properties that contribute to the juice's overall benefits.

Apple cider vinegar is known for its high concentration of acetic acid, which has been shown to have anti-inflammatory and immune-boosting properties. Conversely, Lemon is a great source of vitamin C, which also plays a significant role in supporting the immune system. Honey is a natural sweetener that contains antioxidants and antibacterial properties. At the same time, cinnamon has been shown to have anti-inflammatory properties and may help regulate blood sugar levels.

To make this juice, you'll need to mix two tablespoons of apple cider vinegar with the juice of half a lemon, a tablespoon of honey, and a pinch of cinnamon in a glass of water. Stir well until the honey dissolves completely. Enjoy the tonic on an empty stomach for the best results first thing in the morning.

This tonic can help boost your immune system, reduce inflammation, aid digestion, and promote weight loss. It's a simple and effective way to incorporate these powerful ingredients into your daily routine and reap their many health benefits.

- **Beet Berry Basil Blast: A mix of beets, raspberries, blueberries, basil, and lemon for a powerful antioxidant and anti-inflammatory boost.**

Ingredients:

- 1 medium beet, peeled and chopped
- 1 cup raspberries
- 1 cup blueberries
- 1 handful of fresh basil leaves
- 1 lemon, juiced

Instructions:

1. Wash all fruits and vegetables thoroughly.
2. Add beet, raspberries, blueberries, and basil to a juicer.
3. Juice all ingredients together.
4. Stir in lemon juice.
5. Serve and enjoy your antioxidant and anti-inflammatory boost!

- **Carrot Orange Pineapple Perfection: A combination of carrots, orange, pineapple, and ginger for a delicious and immune-boosting blend.**

Carrot Orange Pineapple Perfection is a delicious and nutrient-dense juice that combines the sweetness of pineapple with the tangy flavor of oranges and the earthiness of carrots. Adding ginger gives it a spicy kick and provides immune-boosting benefits. Pineapple is a good vitamin C and manganese source, while carrots are rich in beta-carotene. This antioxidant converts to vitamin A in the body. Oranges are also high in vitamin C, which helps boost the immune system. At the same time, ginger is a natural anti-inflammatory agent that aids digestion. This juice is a perfect blend of flavors and nutrients, making it an ideal choice for a healthy and refreshing drink.

You will need a juicer or blender to prepare Carrot, Orange Pineapple Perfection juice. Here the recipe:

Ingredients:

- 2-3 medium carrots, washed and chopped
- 1 large orange, peeled and segmented
- 1 cup fresh pineapple chunks
- 1-2 inch piece of fresh ginger, peeled and chopped
- Optional: ice cubes

Instructions:

1. If using a juicer: Juice the carrots, orange, pineapple, and ginger one at a time, in the order listed.
2. If using a blender: Add the chopped carrots, orange segments, pineapple chunks, and ginger to a blender with 1/2 cup of water. Blend until smooth, adding more water as needed to reach your desired consistency.
3. Optional: Add ice cubes to the blender for a cooler, more refreshing drink.
4. Pour the juice into a glass and enjoy!

- **Ginger Lemon Detox: A mix of ginger, lemon, and honey for a powerful immune-boosting and detoxifying blend.**

To prepare a Ginger Lemon Detox juice, you will need:

- 1-inch piece of ginger, peeled and sliced
- 1 lemon, juiced
- 1-2 teaspoons of honey
- 1 cup of water

Instructions:

1. Add the sliced ginger and water to a blender or juicer and blend until smooth.
2. Strain the mixture through a fine-mesh sieve or cheesecloth to remove any pulp.
3. Stir in the lemon juice and honey until well combined.
4. Serve the ginger lemon detox juice immediately over ice, if desired.

Enjoy the refreshing and detoxifying benefits of this delicious juice!

- **Watermelon Mint Cooler:** A combination of watermelon, mint, and lime for a refreshing and immune-boosting blend.

To make a Watermelon Mint Cooler, you will need:

- 2 cups of cubed watermelon
- 1/4 cup of fresh mint leaves
- Juice of 1 lime
- 1/2 cup of water
- Ice cubes

Here are the steps to prepare it:

1. Add the cubed watermelon, fresh mint leaves, lime juice, and water to a blender.
2. Blend until smooth.
3. Add ice cubes to a glass.
4. Pour the watermelon mint mixture over the ice cubes and serve.

You can also strain the mixture through a fine mesh sieve if you prefer a smoother consistency. Enjoy!

- **Carrot Ginger Limeade: A blend of carrots, ginger, lime, and honey for a zesty and immune-boosting juice.**

To prepare Carrot Ginger Limeade, you will need:

- 4 medium-sized carrots, washed and peeled
- 1-inch piece of fresh ginger, peeled and grated
- 2 limes, juiced
- 1 tablespoon of honey
- 2 cups of water

Instructions:

1. Cut the carrots into small pieces and add them to a blender along with grated ginger.
2. Add 2 cups of water and blend until smooth.
3. Strain the juice using a fine mesh strainer or cheesecloth to remove any pulp.
4. Add fresh lime juice and honey to the strained juice and mix well.

5. Serve chilled over ice for a refreshing and immune-boosting drink.

- **Golden Elixir: A mix of turmeric, ginger, carrot, and orange creates a powerful anti-inflammatory and immune-boosting blend.**

To make the Golden Elixir, follow these steps:

Ingredients:

- 1 medium carrot, chopped
- 1-inch piece of fresh ginger, peeled and chopped
- 1-inch piece of fresh turmeric, peeled and chopped
- 1 medium orange, peeled and segmented

Instructions:

1. Add the chopped carrot, ginger, and turmeric to a juicer.
2. Juice the ingredients until smooth.
3. Add the orange segments to the juicer and juice again.
4. Pour the juice into a glass and stir well.
5. Drink immediately for maximum benefits.

This juice is high in antioxidants, anti-inflammatory compounds, and vitamin C, making it a great choice for boosting your immune system and fighting inflammation. It also has a bright, zesty flavor perfect for starting your day or as a midday pick-me-up.

- **Golden Sunrise: A blend of carrots, oranges, ginger, and turmeric for a potent anti-inflammatory and immune-boosting juice.**

Golden Sunrise is a delicious and healthy juice that combines the benefits of carrots, oranges, ginger, and turmeric. Here's how to make it:

Ingredients:

- 4-5 medium-sized carrots, chopped
- 2 oranges, peeled and deseeded
- 1-inch fresh ginger, peeled and chopped
- 1 tsp ground turmeric
- 1 cup of water (or more as needed)

Instructions:

1. In a juicer, juice the carrots, oranges, and ginger together.

2. Add the ground turmeric and mix well.
3. If the juice is too thick, add more water to dilute it to your desired consistency.
4. Pour the juice into a glass and enjoy immediately.

This juice is high in vitamin C, antioxidants, and anti-inflammatory compounds. It's a perfect way to start your day and support your immune system.

- **Sweet Greens: A mix of spinach, kale, green apple, cucumber, and pear for a sweet and nutritious green juice.**

Recipe for Sweet Greens juice:

Ingredients:

- 1 cup spinach
- 1 cup kale
- 1 green apple
- 1 cucumber
- 1 pear

Instructions:

1. Wash all the ingredients properly under running water.
2. Peel the cucumber and remove the core of the pear.
3. Cut the apple, cucumber, and pear into small pieces.
4. Add all the ingredients to a juicer and blend until smooth.
5. Pour the juice into a glass, and serve immediately.

Note: You can add ice cubes to make it more refreshing.

- **Red Radiance: A blend of beets, strawberries, and watermelon for a juice rich in antioxidants and anti-inflammatory compounds.**

Here's a simple recipe for preparing Red Radiance juice:

Ingredients:

- 1 medium-sized beet, washed and peeled
- 1 cup fresh strawberries, washed and hulled
- 2 cups diced watermelon, seeds removed

Instructions:

1. Cut the beet into small pieces.
2. Add all the ingredients into a juicer and juice until smooth.
3. If desired, strain the juice through a fine-mesh sieve to remove any pulp or solids.
4. Serve immediately over ice, if desired. Enjoy your Red Radiance juice!

- **Citrus Zing: A mix of grapefruit, lemon, lime, and ginger for a tangy and refreshing juice that aids in digestion.**

Ingredients:

- 1 grapefruit, peeled and segmented
- 2 lemons, peeled
- 2 limes, peeled
- 1-inch ginger root, peeled

Instructions:

1. Wash all the ingredients thoroughly.
2. Peel and segment the grapefruit.
3. Peel the lemons and limes.
4. Peel the ginger root.

5. Add all the ingredients to a juicer and process until smooth.
6. Pour the juice into a glass and enjoy immediately.

Optional: You can also add a pinch of cayenne pepper for an extra kick.

- **Berry Beet Blast: A mix of beets, blueberries, raspberries, and strawberries for a juice packed with antioxidants and cancer-fighting properties.**

Ingredients:

- 1 medium-sized beet, peeled and chopped
- 1 cup of mixed berries (blueberries, raspberries, and strawberries)
- 1 cup of water

Instructions:

1. Wash and prepare the beet and berries.
2. Add the beet and berries to a blender.
3. Pour in the water.
4. Blend until smooth.

5. Strain the juice through a fine mesh strainer or cheesecloth to remove any pulp.
6. Serve the juice immediately and enjoy!

- **Mango Tango: A mango, ginger, and turmeric blend for tropical and anti-inflammatory juice.**

Here is a simple recipe for Mango Tango juice:

Ingredients:

- 2 ripe mangoes, peeled and chopped
- 1-inch piece of fresh ginger, peeled and grated
- 1 teaspoon turmeric powder
- 1/2 cup water
- Ice cubes (optional)

Instructions:

1. Add the chopped mango, grated ginger, turmeric powder, and water to a blender.
2. Blend the mixture until smooth and well combined.

3. Taste the juice and adjust the sweetness and consistency as desired by adding more water or ice cubes.
4. Pour the juice into glasses and enjoy your delicious and healthy Mango Tango juice.

- **Pink Power: A mix of watermelon, raspberries, and mint for a refreshing, hydrating juice rich in antioxidants.**

Ingredients:

- 2 cups of watermelon chunks
- 1 cup of raspberries
- 5-6 mint leaves
- 1/2 cup of water (optional, for a thinner consistency)

Instructions:

1. Wash all the ingredients thoroughly.
2. Cut the watermelon into small chunks.
3. Place the watermelon, raspberries, and mint leaves in a blender.
4. Blend on high until the mixture is smooth.
5. If the mixture is too thick, add water as needed to reach your desired consistency.
6. Serve the juice chilled and enjoy!

You can also strain the mixture through a fine mesh strainer if you prefer smoother juice.

- **Carrot Topper: A mix of carrots, celery, and apple for a sweet and nutritious juice that supports liver and kidney function**

Ingredients:

- 4 large carrots, washed and peeled
- 2 celery stalks, washed
- 1 apple, cored

Instructions:

1. Cut the carrots, celery, and apple into small pieces that will fit into your juicer.
2. Feed the pieces into the juicer, alternating between the different ingredients.
3. Once all the ingredients have been juiced, stir the mixture to combine the flavors.
4. Pour the juice into a glass and enjoy immediately.

Note: You can adjust the amount of each ingredient to your preference, and you can also add some fresh ginger or lemon juice for an extra kick.

- **Sweet and Sour: A blend of pineapple, lemon, and ginger for a sweet and tangy juice that aids digestion and reduces inflammation.**

Here's the recipe for Sweet and Sour juice:

Ingredients:

- 1 cup of fresh pineapple chunks
- 1 lemon, peeled and sliced
- 1-2 inch piece of fresh ginger, peeled and chopped
- 1 tablespoon of honey (optional)

Instructions:

1. Wash and prepare all the ingredients.
2. Juice the pineapple, lemon, and ginger using a juicer.
3. If desired, stir in honey until well combined.
4. Serve chilled over ice and enjoy!

- **Green Glow:** A mix of spinach, cucumber, celery, green apple, and lemon for a nutrient-dense and alkalizing juice that promotes detoxification.

To prepare Green Glow juice, follow these steps:

Ingredients:

- 2 cups fresh spinach
- 1 medium cucumber
- 2 celery stalks
- 1 green apple
- 1/2 lemon, juiced

Instructions:

1. Wash all the ingredients thoroughly.
2. Cut the cucumber and green apple into smaller pieces so they can fit into your juicer.
3. Feed the spinach, cucumber, celery, and green apple into a juicer.
4. Once all the ingredients have been juiced, pour the juice into a glass.
5. Squeeze half a lemon into the juice and stir well.

6. Serve immediately and enjoy your nutrient-dense and alkalizing Green Glow juice.

- **Purple Passion: A blend of blueberries, blackberries, strawberries, and raspberries for a juice rich in antioxidants and cancer-fighting properties**

Ingredients:

- 1 cup blueberries
- 1 cup blackberries
- 1 cup strawberries
- 1 cup raspberries
- 1 cup water

Instructions:

1. Wash all the berries and pat them dry with a paper towel.
2. Add the berries to a blender along with the water.
3. Blend until smooth and well combined.

4. If the juice is too thick, you can add more water until you reach the desired consistency.
5. Pour the juice into a glass and enjoy immediately.

Note: You can also add a sweetener of your choice if you prefer a sweeter juice. Honey or agave syrup would be good options.

- **Kiwi Kiss: A mix of kiwi, lime, and honey for a refreshing and immune-boosting juice that supports healthy digestion and aids in nutrient absorption.**

To prepare Kiwi Kiss juice, you will need:

- 2 kiwis, peeled and chopped
- 1 lime, juiced
- 1-2 teaspoons honey (optional)
- 1/2 cup of water

Instructions:

1. Add the chopped kiwi and lime juice to a blender.
2. Blend until smooth.

3. If desired, add honey and water to the blender and blend until well combined.
4. Pour the juice into a glass and enjoy.

- **Red Reboot: A blend of beets, carrots, ginger, and lemon for a juice that promotes liver function and reduces inflammation.**

Ingredients:

- 1 medium beet, chopped
- 2 medium carrots, chopped
- 1-inch piece of fresh ginger, peeled and chopped
- 1 lemon, juiced

Directions:

1. Wash and prepare all the ingredients.
2. Run the beet, carrots, and ginger through a juicer, collecting the juice in a large glass or pitcher.
3. Stir in the freshly squeezed lemon juice.
4. Serve the juice immediately over ice, or store it in an airtight container in the refrigerator for up to 24 hours.

Enjoy your Red Reboot juice!

- **Carrot Craze: A mix of carrots, oranges, and ginger for a sweet and spicy juice that supports healthy digestion and immune function**

To prepare Carrot Craze juice, you will need the following **ingredients:**

- 4-5 medium-sized carrots
- 2 oranges
- 1-inch piece of fresh ginger

Instructions:

1. Wash the carrots, oranges, and ginger properly.
2. Peel the oranges and cut them into small pieces.
3. Cut the carrots into small pieces.
4. Peel the ginger and chop it into small pieces.
5. Put all the ingredients into a juicer.
6. Blend until smooth and serve immediately.

Enjoy your delicious and nutritious Carrot Craze juice!

- **Tropical Twist: A pineapple, mango, and papaya blend for a tropical and anti-inflammatory juice rich in enzymes and vitamins.**

To make Tropical Twist juice, you will need:

- 1 cup fresh pineapple chunks
- 1 cup fresh mango chunks
- 1 cup fresh papaya chunks

Instructions:

1. Wash all the fruits properly and chop them into small chunks.
2. Add the chopped fruits to the juicer.
3. Turn on the juicer and let it blend the fruits.
4. Once done, pour the juice into a glass.
5. You can add ice if you want a cold drink.
6. Enjoy your Tropical Twist juice!

- **Berry Beautiful: A mix of strawberries, raspberries, blackberries, and mint for a refreshing and antioxidant-rich juice that supports healthy skin and digestion**

Ingredients:

- 1 cup strawberries
- 1 cup raspberries
- 1 cup blackberries
- 5-6 mint leaves
- 1/2 cup water

Instructions:

1. Rinse all the berries and mint leaves under cold water.
2. Remove the stems from the strawberries.
3. Add the berries and mint leaves to a blender or juicer.
4. Pour in the water and blend or juice until smooth.
5. Strain the juice through a fine mesh strainer to remove any seeds or pulp, if desired.
6. Serve the juice immediately over ice and enjoy!

- **Lemon Limeade: A mix of lemon, lime, honey, and water for a refreshing and alkalizing juice that supports detoxification and digestion**

To prepare Lemon Limeade juice, follow these steps:

Ingredients:

- 2 lemons
- 2 limes
- 2 tablespoons honey
- 4 cups water

Instructions:

1. Juice the lemons and limes into a pitcher.
2. Add honey and water to the pitcher and stir until the honey dissolves.
3. Serve over ice and enjoy your refreshing and alkalizing Lemon Limeade juice.

- **Grapefruit Ginger: A blend of grapefruit, ginger, and honey for a tangy and anti-inflammatory juice that supports immune function**

Grapefruit Ginger juice can provide several benefits to cancer patients. Grapefruit is a rich source of antioxidants, vitamins, and minerals that help protect cells from damage caused by free radicals. Ginger contains compounds with anti-inflammatory properties that can help reduce inflammation and may have a protective effect against cancer. Additionally, ginger can help alleviate nausea and vomiting, common side effects of cancer treatment. Honey has antioxidant and anti-inflammatory properties and can help soothe a sore throat.

To prepare Grapefruit Ginger juice, follow these steps:

Ingredients:

- 1 large grapefruit, peeled and deseeded
- 1-inch piece of fresh ginger, peeled
- 1-2 teaspoons honey (optional)
- 1/2 cup water

Instructions:

1. Cut the grapefruit into small pieces and place them in a blender.
2. Grate the ginger and add it to the blender.

3. Add honey and water to the blender.
4. Blend all the ingredients together until smooth.
5. Pour the juice through a strainer to remove any pulp or ginger fibers.
6. Serve the juice chilled or over ice.

- **Orange Oasis: A mix of oranges, carrots, and turmeric for a refreshing and immune-boosting juice that supports healthy skin and digestion**

Ingredients:

- 4 oranges, peeled
- 4 large carrots, peeled and chopped
- 1/2 inch pieces of fresh turmeric root, peeled
- Ice (optional)

Instructions:

1. Wash and prep the oranges, carrots, and turmeric.
2. Juice the oranges, carrots, and turmeric.
3. If desired, pour the juice over ice and serve immediately.

Enjoy your refreshing and immune-boosting Orange Oasis juice!

- **Kale Crush: A blend of kale, cucumber, celery, and lemon for a nutrient-dense and alkalizing juice that supports detoxification and digestion.**

Kale is a cruciferous vegetable that contains compounds that have been shown to have anti-cancer properties. It is also a rich source of vitamins and minerals that support the immune system, which can be compromised in cancer patients. Cucumbers and celery are also hydrating vegetables high in antioxidants and anti-inflammatory compounds, which can help reduce cancer risk and support overall health.

To prepare Kale Crush, you will need the following ingredients:

- 2 cups of chopped kale leaves
- 1 medium cucumber, chopped
- 2 celery stalks, chopped
- 1 lemon, juiced

Directions:

1. Wash and chop all the ingredients.
2. Add the kale, cucumber, and celery to a juicer and extract the juice.
3. Squeeze the juice of one lemon into the mixture and stir.
4. Serve immediately and enjoy.

Note: If you do not have a juicer, you can also blend the ingredients with a little bit of water and then strain the mixture through a fine-mesh strainer or cheesecloth to remove any pulp.

- **Red Rejuvenator: A mix of beets, strawberries, and ginger for a juice rich in antioxidants and anti-inflammatory compounds that promotes healthy blood flow.**

Red Rejuvenator is a juice that combines beets, strawberries, and ginger and is packed with antioxidants and anti-inflammatory compounds. The juice helps in promoting healthy blood flow, which can be beneficial for cancer patients.

Here's a simple recipe to make Red Rejuvenator at home:

Ingredients:

- 1 medium-sized beet, peeled and chopped
- 1 cup of fresh strawberries, hulled and chopped
- 1-inch piece of fresh ginger, peeled and grated
- 1 cup of water

Instructions:

1. Add the chopped beets, strawberries, and grated ginger to a blender or juicer.
2. Add a cup of water and blend until smooth.
3. Strain the juice through a fine-mesh sieve or a cheesecloth.
4. Serve the juice immediately over ice.

Note: If the juice is too thick, you can add more water to thin it out to your desired consistency.

- **Sweet Sunshine: A blend of carrots, oranges, and pineapple for a sweet and tangy juice that supports healthy digestion and immune function**

To prepare Sweet Sunshine juice, follow these steps to get your sweet sunshine:

Ingredients:

- 4 medium carrots, washed and peeled
- 2 medium oranges, peeled and segmented
- 1 cup of chopped pineapple

Instructions:

1. Cut the carrots into small pieces and put them into a juicer.
2. Add the orange segments to the juicer and juice them along with the carrots.
3. Add the chopped pineapple to the juicer and juice it along with the carrot and orange juice.
4. Stir the juice well and serve immediately.

Enjoy your sweet and tangy Sweet Sunshine juice!

- **Cucumber Cooler: A mix of cucumber, lime, and mint for a refreshing, hydrating juice that supports healthy skin and digestion**

To prepare Cucumber Cooler:

Ingredients:

- 1 large cucumber
- 1 lime
- a handful of fresh mint leaves
- 1 cup of water

Instructions:

1. Wash the cucumber and chop it into small pieces.
2. Cut the lime into wedges.
3. Add the cucumber pieces, lime wedges, and mint leaves to a blender.
4. Add a cup of water to the blender.
5. Blend the mixture until it is smooth.
6. Pour the mixture through a strainer to remove any solids.
7. Serve the juice over ice and garnish with additional mint leaves, if desired.

- **Ginger Green: A blend of spinach, kale, green apple, ginger, and lemon for a nutrient-dense and anti-inflammatory juice that supports healthy digestion and immune function**

The Ginger Green juice is a great source of nutrients and anti-inflammatory compounds.

Ingredients:

- 2 cups of spinach
- 2 cups of kale
- 1 green apple
- 1-inch piece of fresh ginger
- 1 lemon, juiced

Instructions:

1. Wash all the ingredients thoroughly.
2. Cut the apple into chunks and remove the stem.
3. Peel the ginger and cut it into small pieces.
4. Add the spinach, kale, apple, ginger, and lemon juice to a juicer.
5. Juice all the ingredients together.
6. Pour the juice into a glass and enjoy!

- **Purple Powerhouse: A mix of blueberries, blackberries, raspberries, and kale for a juice rich in antioxidants and anti-inflammatory compounds that promotes healthy brain function and helps fight against cancer.**

Purple Powerhouse juice provides numerous benefits to cancer patients due to its high antioxidant and anti-inflammatory content. The berries in the juice, such as blueberries, blackberries, and raspberries, are rich in polyphenols, which have been shown to have anticancer effects. Kale, on the other hand, is rich in vitamins, minerals, and phytochemicals that can help reduce inflammation and oxidative stress in the body, which can contribute to cancer development.

To prepare Purple Powerhouse juice, blend a handful of **kale** with a cup of **mixed berries** (blueberries, blackberries, and raspberries), along with some **water** or **coconut water.** You can also add some **lemon juice** for extra flavor and vitamin C. Blend all the ingredients until smooth, and enjoy your antioxidant-rich juice.

- **Immunity Booster: A blend of kiwi, lemon, orange, and spinach to strengthen the immune system and fight off cancer cells**

Immunity Booster juice benefits cancer patients by providing essential nutrients that help to support the immune system and fight against cancer cells. The kiwi and citrus fruits are rich in vitamin C, which is an antioxidant that helps to protect the body against free radicals that can cause cancer. Spinach is rich in chlorophyll, which can help neutralize carcinogens in the body. It is also high in iron, important for maintaining healthy blood cells.

To prepare the Immunity Booster juice, follow these steps:

1. Peel and slice 2 kiwis.
2. Peel and segment 1 orange.
3. Squeeze the juice of 1 lemon.
4. Wash and chop 2 cups of spinach leaves.
5. Add all the ingredients to a blender and blend until smooth.
6. If the mixture is too thick, add a splash of water to thin it out.
7. Pour the juice into a glass and enjoy immediately.

- **Spicy Green: A mix of green apple, cucumber, jalapeno, and cilantro to reduce inflammation and provide a kick of heat**

Spicy Green is a juice blend of green apples, cucumber, jalapeno, and cilantro. This juice is known for its anti-inflammatory properties and ability to aid digestion. The jalapeno pepper adds a spicy kick, while the cucumber and apple help to balance the heat with their refreshing flavors. Cilantro is known for its detoxifying properties, making this juice a great option for those looking to cleanse their body. To prepare, blend all the ingredients in a juicer or high-speed blender and serve over ice. You can adjust the amount of jalapeno to your desired level of spiciness.

- **Purple Love: A blend of purple cabbage, blackberries, and ginger for a powerful antioxidant boost.**

Ingredients:

- 1 cup purple cabbage
- 1/2 cup blackberries
- 1/2 inch ginger root
- 1/2 cup water

Instructions:

1. Wash and chop the purple cabbage and ginger root into small pieces.
2. Add the cabbage, blackberries, and ginger to a blender or juicer.
3. Add the water and blend until smooth.
4. Strain the juice through a fine-mesh strainer or cheesecloth to remove any pulp.
5. Serve the juice immediately or store it in an airtight container in the refrigerator for up to 2 days.

Enjoy your Purple Love juice!

- **Citrus Splash: A mix of grapefruit, lime, lemon, and mint to aid in digestion and provide a dose of vitamin C**

Ingredients:

- 1 grapefruit
- 2 limes
- 2 lemons
- A handful of fresh mint leaves
- Water (optional)

Instructions:

1. Cut the grapefruit, limes, and lemons into wedges and remove any seeds.
2. Place the citrus wedges and mint leaves in a blender and blend until smooth.
3. If the mixture is too thick, add a small amount of water to thin it out.
4. Pour the juice through a strainer to remove any pulp or seeds.
5. Serve over ice and enjoy!

This recipe makes about 2-3 servings. You can adjust the amount of mint and water to your liking.

- **Orange Creamsicle: A blend of orange, vanilla, and coconut milk for a creamy and delicious treat high in antioxidants**

To prepare Orange Creamsicle juice, you will need:

- 2 medium oranges
- 1/2 cup coconut milk
- 1/2 teaspoon vanilla extract

Instructions:

1. Peel and segment the oranges and place them in a blender.
2. Add the coconut milk and vanilla extract to the blender.
3. Blend the ingredients until smooth and creamy.
4. Pour the juice into a glass and enjoy immediately.

Optional: You can add ice to make it more refreshing. You can also use other types of milk, such as almond or soy milk, instead of coconut milk.

- **Green Goddess: A mix of kale, parsley, celery, and pear to detoxify the body and provide a nutrient-dense juice**

Here is a simple recipe for Green Goddess juice:

Ingredients:

- 2 cups kale leaves
- 1 bunch parsley
- 2 stalks celery
- 1 pear

Instructions:

1. Rinse all ingredients well.
2. Cut the kale, parsley, celery, and pear into pieces that will fit into your juicer.
3. Run all ingredients through a juicer.
4. Pour the juice into a glass and enjoy!

This juice is packed with nutrients, including vitamins A, C, and K, and minerals like potassium and magnesium. It's also great for detoxification and supporting healthy digestion.

- **Beet It: A blend of beets, carrots, and ginger to reduce inflammation and provide a dose of vitamins and minerals**

Ingredients:

- 1 medium beet, peeled and chopped
- 2 medium carrots, peeled and chopped
- 1/2 inch piece of ginger, peeled
- 1 cup of water

Instructions:

1. Add the chopped beet, carrots, and ginger to a blender.
2. Pour in 1 cup of water.

3. Blend at high speed until the mixture is smooth.
4. Strain the mixture through a fine-mesh strainer to remove any solids.
5. Serve the juice immediately or store it in the refrigerator for up to 24 hours.

Enjoy your anti-inflammatory and nutrient-dense "Beet It" juice!

- **Melon Medley: A mix of watermelon, honeydew, and mint for a refreshing and hydrating juice that is also high in antioxidants**

To prepare Melon Medley juice, follow these steps:

Ingredients:

- 2 cups chopped watermelon
- 2 cups chopped honeydew melon
- 1/4 cup fresh mint leaves
- 1/2 cup water (optional)

Instructions:

1. Wash and chop the watermelon and honeydew melon into small pieces.
2. Rinse the mint leaves.
3. Add the watermelon, honeydew melon, and mint leaves to a blender.
4. If necessary, add a bit of water to help with blending.
5. Blend the ingredients until smooth.
6. Pour the juice into a glass and serve chilled. Enjoy!

Note: You can adjust the number of mint leaves to your liking, depending on how strong you want the mint flavor to be.

- **Lemon Ginger Zing: A blend of lemon, ginger, and apple cider vinegar to aid in digestion and reduce inflammation**

To prepare Lemon Ginger Zing juice, follow these steps:

Ingredients:

- 1 lemon, peeled and quartered
- 1-inch piece of ginger, peeled
- 1 tablespoon apple cider vinegar
- 1 cup of water

- Ice cubes

Instructions:

1. In a juicer, juice the lemon and ginger together.
2. In a glass, mix the lemon and ginger juice with apple cider vinegar and water.
3. Add ice cubes and stir well.
4. Enjoy immediately.

Note: If you don't have a juicer, you can blend the lemon and ginger in a blender and then strain the mixture through a fine-mesh sieve to remove any pulp before mixing it with apple cider vinegar and water.

- **Turmeric Tango: A turmeric, orange, and pineapple mix to reduce inflammation and boost antioxidants**

Ingredients:

- 2 oranges, peeled and segmented
- 1/2 cup pineapple chunks
- 1 tsp grated fresh turmeric root
- 1 cup water

Directions:

1. Add the oranges, pineapple, and turmeric to a blender and blend until smooth.
2. Add water to thin out the juice to your desired consistency and blend again.
3. Pour the juice into a glass and enjoy immediately.

Note: If you don't have fresh turmeric root, you can substitute it with 1/2 tsp of ground turmeric. You can also add a pinch of black pepper to the juice to enhance the absorption of the turmeric.

- **Immune Boost: A blend of orange, ginger, and turmeric to support the immune system and reduce inflammation**

Immune Boost juice is great for supporting the immune system and reducing inflammation. Oranges are high in vitamin C, which helps to boost the immune system. At the same time, ginger and turmeric have anti-inflammatory properties that can help to reduce inflammation in the body.

To make Immune Boost juice, you will need:

- 2 oranges, peeled and segmented
- 1 inch of fresh ginger root, peeled
- 1 inch of fresh turmeric root, peeled
- 1/2 cup of water

Instructions:

1. Add the oranges, ginger, and turmeric to a juicer and juice until smooth.
2. Add the water to the juice and stir to combine.
3. Serve the juice immediately over ice.

Enjoy your delicious and immune-boosting juice!

- **Sunset Glow: A mix of carrot, grapefruit, and ginger for a delicious and nutritious juice**

Here's the recipe for Sunset Glow:

Ingredients:

- 4 medium carrots
- 1 grapefruit
- 1-inch pieces of fresh ginger

Instructions:

1. Wash and peel the carrots, then cut them into smaller pieces that will fit into your juicer.
2. Cut the grapefruit in half and remove any seeds.
3. Peel the ginger and cut it into smaller pieces.
4. Feed the carrots, grapefruit, and ginger through your juicer, alternating between the ingredients.
5. Stir the juice well and pour it into a glass.
6. Enjoy your delicious and nutritious Sunset Glow juice!

- **Purple Haze: A blend of blueberries, raspberries, and kale, rich in antioxidants and anti-inflammatory compounds**

Ingredients:
- 1 cup blueberries
- 1 cup raspberries
- 1 cup kale leaves, washed and chopped
- 1 cup water

Instructions:

1. Rinse the blueberries and raspberries and add them to a blender.
2. Add the chopped kale leaves to the blender as well.
3. Pour in one cup of water.
4. Blend the ingredients on high speed until smooth and creamy.
5. Pour the juice into a glass and enjoy!

Note: If you prefer a sweeter juice, you can add a small amount of honey or maple syrup to taste.

- **The Ultimate Detox: A mix of cucumber, celery, kale, and lemon for a powerful detoxifying juice.**

Ingredients:

- 1 cucumber
- 2 celery stalks
- 2 kale leaves
- 1/2 lemon, juiced

Instructions:

1. Wash all the ingredients thoroughly.

2. Cut the cucumber, celery, and kale into smaller pieces that will fit into your juicer.
3. Juice all the ingredients, starting with the cucumber, then celery, followed by the kale.
4. Squeeze the juice of half a lemon into the mixture and stir.
5. Enjoy your Ultimate Detox juice immediately.

Note: You can adjust the amount of lemon juice to your taste preference. If you prefer a sweeter taste, you can add an apple or pear to the mix.

- **Pineapple Ginger Blast: A mix of pineapple, ginger, and mint to aid digestion and reduce inflammation.**

Ingredients:

- 1 cup pineapple chunks
- 1-inch piece of ginger, peeled and chopped
- A handful of fresh mint leaves
- 1 cup water

Instructions:

1. Add the pineapple, ginger, and mint leaves to a blender.
2. Pour in the water and blend until smooth.
3. Strain the juice through a fine mesh strainer to remove any solids.
4. Serve chilled and enjoy!

- **Lemon Berry Blast: A blend of lemon, blueberries, and strawberries for a refreshing and immune-boosting juice**

Ingredients:

- 1 lemon, peeled and seeded
- 1 cup of blueberries
- 1 cup of strawberries
- 1 cup of water
- **Optional:** honey or maple syrup for sweetness

Instructions:

1. Add the lemon, blueberries, strawberries, and water to a blender.
2. Blend at high speed until the mixture is smooth and well-combined.
3. Taste the mixture and add honey or maple syrup if desired.

4. Pour the juice into a glass and enjoy immediately.

This juice is packed with vitamin C, antioxidants, and anti-inflammatory compounds from berries and lemon, which can help boost your immune system and support healthy skin.

- **Turmeric Tonic: A mix of turmeric, ginger, and lemon for a powerful anti-inflammatory and immune-boosting juice**

Turmeric Tonic is a potent anti-inflammatory and immune-boosting juice. Here's the recipe:

Ingredients:

- 2 inches fresh turmeric root
- 1-inch fresh ginger root
- 1 lemon, peeled
- 1 apple, cored
- 1/4 tsp black pepper
- 1/4 cup water

Instructions:

1. Peel and chop the turmeric and ginger.

2. Add the turmeric, ginger, lemon, apple, black pepper, and water to a blender.
3. Blend until smooth.
4. Strain the juice through a fine-mesh strainer or nut milk bag to remove any pulp.
5. Serve immediately and enjoy the benefits of this powerful tonic.

- **Berry Beet Blast: A blend of beets, raspberries, and blueberries for a delicious and nutrient-packed juice**

Beets are high in antioxidants and help reduce inflammation. At the same time, raspberries and blueberries are also rich in antioxidants and can support brain health. Here's the Berry Beet Blast recipe:

Ingredients:

- 1 medium beet, peeled and chopped
- 1 cup raspberries
- 1 cup blueberries
- 1/2 cup water

Directions:

1. Add the chopped beet, raspberries, blueberries, and water to a blender.
2. Blend at high speed until the mixture is smooth and well combined.
3. Pour the juice through a fine mesh strainer to remove any pulp or seeds, if desired.
4. Serve immediately and enjoy!

- **Minty Melon: A mix of watermelon, mint, and lime for a refreshing and hydrating juice**

Watermelon is a great source of hydration and also provides vitamins and minerals like vitamin C and potassium. Mint can aid in digestion and provide a fresh flavor, while lime adds a tangy kick of vitamin C. Enjoy!

Recipe for Minty Melon juice:

Ingredients:

- 2 cups chopped watermelon
- 1 cup chopped honeydew melon
- 1-2 sprigs of fresh mint leaves
- 1 lime, juiced

Instructions:

1. Add the watermelon, honeydew melon, and mint leaves to a blender.
2. Squeeze the juice of one lime over the top of the ingredients.
3. Blend all the ingredients until smooth.
4. Strain the mixture using a fine-mesh strainer if desired.
5. Pour the juice into glasses and serve chilled.

Enjoy your refreshing and hydrating Minty Melon juice!

- **Green Goddess: A blend of spinach, cucumber, celery, green apple, and lemon for a nutrient-dense and alkalizing juice**

Green Goddess is a nutritious and alkalizing juice that provides a variety of vitamins, minerals, and antioxidants. Here's the recipe:

Ingredients:

- 2 cups spinach
- 1 cucumber
- 2 celery stalks
- 1 green apple

- 1/2 lemon, juiced

Instructions:

1. Wash all the ingredients thoroughly.
2. Cut the cucumber and apple into small pieces.
3. Add all ingredients into a juicer and blend well.
4. Pour the juice into a glass and enjoy immediately.

This juice is packed with nutrients and can be a great addition to a healthy diet.

- **Sunrise Bliss: A blend of oranges, carrots, and turmeric for a powerful dose of vitamin C and anti-inflammatory benefits**

The oranges and carrots provide a good source of vitamin C and beta-carotene, while turmeric adds anti-inflammatory benefits due to its active ingredient, curcumin. Here's how you can make Sunrise Bliss:

Ingredients:

- 4 medium oranges, peeled
- 4 medium carrots, peeled
- 1-inch piece of fresh turmeric root, peeled
- Ice cubes (optional)

Instructions:

1. Cut the oranges and carrots into small pieces that will fit into your juicer chute.
2. Add the orange, carrot, and turmeric pieces into the juicer.
3. Juice until all ingredients are fully juiced.
4. Serve over ice, if desired.
5. Enjoy your Sunrise Bliss!

- **Ginger Lime Cooler: A mix of ginger, lime, and cucumber for a refreshing and invigorating drink that aids digestion and reduces inflammation**

To prepare Ginger Lime Cooler juice, follow these steps:

Ingredients:

- 1 large cucumber
- 1 lime
- 2 inches of fresh ginger root

Instructions:

1. Peel the cucumber and cut it into small pieces.
2. Peel the ginger root and cut it into small pieces.
3. Juice the cucumber and ginger using a juicer.
4. Squeeze the lime into the juice and stir well.
5. Add ice cubes if desired.
6. Serve immediately and enjoy your refreshing Ginger Lime Cooler!

- **Ruby Red Rejuvenator: A combination of beets, strawberries, and raspberries for a high-antioxidant drink that helps to cleanse the blood and support the immune system**

Beets are a great source of antioxidants and have been shown to support healthy blood pressure and cardiovascular health. Strawberries and raspberries are also high in antioxidants, vitamin C, and fiber. Drinking this juice regularly could help detoxify, immunity, and overall health.

Ruby Red Rejuvenator will benefit you as it is a rich source of antioxidants that helps to reduce oxidative stress in the body. Oxidative stress can lead to cell damage, contributing to cancer development. Additionally, beets are rich in betalains, which have been shown to have anti-cancer properties.

To prepare the Ruby Red Rejuvenator, you will need:

- 1 medium-sized beet, peeled and chopped
- 1 cup of strawberries
- 1 cup of raspberries
- Water (optional)

Instructions:

1. Wash and chop the beet into small pieces.
2. Add the beet, strawberries, and raspberries to a juicer or blender.
3. Blend the ingredients until smooth. If the mixture is too thick, add some water to thin it out.
4. Pour the juice into a glass and serve immediately.

- **Pineapple Green Goddess: A mix of pineapple, kale, and cucumber makes a sweet and refreshing drink rich in nutrients and helps to alkalize the body.**

Pineapple Green Goddess is a nutritious juice that may benefit cancer patients in several ways. Pineapple contains bromelain, an enzyme that has anti-inflammatory properties and may help to reduce swelling and inflammation associated with cancer treatment. Kale is a cruciferous vegetable that contains compounds called glucosinolates, which have been shown to have anti-cancer properties. Cucumber is also a good source of antioxidants. It has anti-inflammatory properties, which can help to reduce oxidative stress and inflammation in the body.

To prepare Pineapple Green Goddess, you will need:

- 2 cups chopped fresh pineapple
- 2 cups chopped kale
- 1 large cucumber, chopped

Directions

1. Wash and prepare the ingredients.

2. Put all the ingredients in a juicer and process until smooth.

3. If you don't have a juicer, you can also blend the ingredients in a blender and then strain the juice through a fine mesh strainer or cheesecloth.

Enjoy the juice immediately or store it in an airtight container in the refrigerator for up to 24 hours.

- **Minty Melon Medley: A blend of watermelon, honeydew, and mint for a hydrating and cooling drink that supports the immune system and aids digestion**

Minty Melon Medley is a refreshing drink that can benefit cancer patients in several ways. Watermelon and honeydew are rich in vitamins A and C, which are essential for a healthy immune system. Additionally, these melons are high in water content, which can help cancer patients stay hydrated during treatment. The addition of mint can also help with digestion and reduce inflammation.

To prepare the Minty Melon Medley, follow these steps:

Ingredients:

- 2 cups watermelon, cubed
- 2 cups honeydew, cubed
- 1/4 cup fresh mint leaves
- Ice cubes

Instructions:

1. Add watermelon, honeydew, and mint leaves to a blender.
2. Blend until smooth.
3. If the mixture is too thick, add a little water or ice cubes to thin it out.
4. Pour the mixture into a glass and add ice cubes if desired.
5. Enjoy your Minty Melon Medley!

- **Pineapple Green Goddess: A mix of pineapple, kale, and cucumber for a sweet and refreshing drink that is rich in nutrients and helps to alkalize the body.**

Ingredients:

- 1 cup chopped kale leaves
- 1 cup chopped cucumber
- 1 cup chopped fresh pineapple

Instructions:

1. Wash and chop the kale, cucumber, and pineapple into small pieces.
2. Add all the ingredients to a blender or juicer.
3. Blend until smooth.
4. Pour the mixture into a glass and enjoy!

Benefits for you:

- Kale is a cruciferous vegetable that contains cancer-fighting compounds.
- Pineapple contains an enzyme called bromelain, which has been shown to have anti-inflammatory and anti-cancer properties.
- Cucumber is high in antioxidants and can help to reduce inflammation in the body.
- This juice is rich in nutrients and helps to alkalize the body, which can be beneficial for cancer patients.

- **Spicy Carrot Kick: A mix of carrots, ginger, and cayenne pepper for a spicy and energizing drink that helps to reduce inflammation and boost the metabolism**

The Spicy Carrot Kick juice contains carrots rich in beta-carotene and vitamin A, which have been shown to have anti-cancer properties. Ginger and cayenne pepper have anti-inflammatory effects and may help to boost the immune system. The preparation mode is to juice 5-6 large carrots, 1-2 inches of fresh ginger root, and a pinch of cayenne pepper together. Serve over ice, and enjoy!

- **Cherry Berry Blast: A combination of cherries, blueberries, and raspberries for a delicious and antioxidant-rich drink that supports the immune system and helps to fight cancer**

Cherries, blueberries, and raspberries are all rich in antioxidants, which can help to protect the body from damage caused by harmful molecules called free radicals. Free radicals can contribute

211

to cancer development, so consuming antioxidant-rich foods and drinks like the Cherry Berry Blast may help reduce the risk of cancer.

To make the Cherry Berry Blast, blend 1 cup of pitted cherries, 1 cup of blueberries, and 1 cup of raspberries until smooth. If the mixture is too thick, add some water to thin it out. Enjoy immediately for maximum nutritional benefits.

- **Green Tea Infusion: A blend of green tea, lemon, and honey for a refreshing and antioxidant-rich drink that helps to reduce inflammation and support the immune system.**

Green tea is known for its antioxidant properties, which help to protect cells and reduce inflammation in the body. Adding lemon and honey boosts vitamin C and anti-inflammatory compounds, making it a great drink for supporting the immune system. Here's a recipe for a Green Tea Infusion:

Ingredients:

- 2 green tea bags
- 1 lemon, sliced

- 2 tablespoons of honey
- 4 cups of water
- Ice cubes

Instructions:

1. Bring 4 cups of water to a boil in a pot.
2. Remove the pot from heat and add 2 green tea bags. Steep for 5 minutes.
3. Remove the tea bags and let the tea cool to room temperature.
4. Add sliced lemon and honey to the tea.
5. Stir until the honey dissolves.
6. Pour the mixture into a pitcher and chill in the refrigerator.
7. Serve with ice cubes and enjoy!

- **Turmeric Sunshine: A mix of turmeric, oranges, and carrots for a sunny and anti-inflammatory drink that helps to boost the immune system and fight cancer**

Turmeric Sunshine is a delicious and nutritious drink with numerous health benefits. The mix of turmeric, oranges, and carrots creates a sunny, vibrant drink rich in antioxidants and anti-inflammatory compounds. Turmeric contains a powerful antioxidant called curcumin, which has been shown to have anti-cancer properties and help to reduce inflammation in the body.

Oranges are a great source of vitamin C, which is important for a healthy immune system. Carrots are packed with beta-carotene, which the body converts into vitamin A for healthy skin, vision, and immune function.

To prepare Turmeric Sunshine, you will need:

- 1 orange, peeled and segmented
- 2 medium-sized carrots, peeled and chopped
- 1 tsp grated turmeric root (or 1/2 tsp ground turmeric)
- 1 cup of water
- **Optional:** honey or maple syrup to sweeten

Preparation

1. Add the orange segments, chopped carrots, and grated turmeric to a blender.
2. Add a cup of water and blend until smooth.

3. Taste and add honey or maple syrup if desired.
4. Pour into a glass and enjoy immediately.

You can also add ice cubes or frozen fruit to the blender to make a chilled or thicker drink.

- **Golden Carrot Elixir: A combination of carrots, apples, and turmeric for a sweet and spicy drink that is rich in antioxidants and helps to reduce inflammation.**

Carrots are an excellent source of beta-carotene, which the body converts into vitamin A, a powerful antioxidant. Apples are also rich in antioxidants and fiber, which can help improve digestion and promote heart health. Turmeric contains curcumin, a compound with anti-inflammatory properties that may also have anticancer effects. Here's a recipe for Golden Carrot Elixir:

Ingredients:

- 3 medium carrots, peeled and chopped
- 2 medium apples, cored and chopped

- 1-inch piece of fresh turmeric, peeled and chopped
- 1/2-inch piece of fresh ginger, peeled and chopped
- 1/2 lemon, juiced

Instructions:

1. Add the carrots, apples, turmeric, and ginger to a juicer and juice.
2. Pour the juice into a glass and stir in the lemon juice.
3. Enjoy immediately.

- **Radiant Glow: A mix of carrots, oranges, and ginger for a high-vitamin C drink that supports healthy skin and boosts the immune system.**

Radiant Glow is a delicious and nutritious juice that is perfect for those looking to improve the health and appearance of their skin, while also boosting their immune system. This juice is made with a combination of carrots, oranges, and ginger, which are all rich in vitamin C and other antioxidants.

To make Radiant Glow, you will need:

- 4 medium carrots
- 2 large oranges
- 1-inch piece of ginger

Instructions:

1. Wash and chop the carrots into small pieces.
2. Peel the oranges and chop them into quarters.
3. Peel the ginger and chop it into small pieces.
4. Add the chopped carrots, oranges, and ginger to a juicer.
5. Juice the ingredients until smooth and well combined.
6. Pour the juice into a glass and enjoy immediately.

The high levels of vitamin C in this juice help to support collagen production, which is essential for healthy skin. Additionally, the antioxidants in carrots and oranges help to protect the skin from damage caused by free radicals. In contrast, ginger helps to reduce inflammation throughout the body and boost the immune system.

Overall, Radiant Glow is a delicious and nutritious juice that can help improve your skin's health and appearance while supporting your immune system.

- **Sunset Serenity: A combination of papaya, oranges, and turmeric for a refreshing, immune-boosting drink that helps reduce inflammation.**

This vibrant drink is packed with nutrients that are essential for maintaining good health, particularly for cancer patients.

Papaya is rich in vitamins A, C, and E, as well as antioxidants that help to protect cells from damage caused by free radicals. Oranges are an excellent source of vitamin C, which is important for supporting the immune system and promoting healthy skin. Turmeric contains curcumin, a powerful anti-inflammatory compound that can help to reduce inflammation throughout the body.

To prepare Sunset Serenity, simply blend 1 cup of chopped papaya, 2 oranges (peeled and seeded), and 1 teaspoon of ground turmeric until smooth. You can also add a few ice cubes or a splash of water to adjust the consistency to your liking.

Enjoy this delicious and nutritious drink as a refreshing snack or a healthy addition to your breakfast routine. It's sure to leave you feeling energized and radiant!

- **Emerald Elixir: A mix of cucumber, spinach, green apple, and lime for a hydrating and alkalizing drink that supports overall health and well-being.**

Emerald Elixir Recipe:

Ingredients:

- 1 medium cucumber
- 2 cups of spinach
- 1 green apple
- 1 lime, juiced

Instructions:

1. Wash all the ingredients thoroughly.
2. Cut the cucumber and green apple into small pieces.

3. Put the cucumber, spinach, and green apple into a juicer and juice until smooth.
4. Pour the juice into a glass and stir in the lime juice.
5. Serve and enjoy!

Benefits:

This juice is rich in vitamins and minerals that support overall health and well-being. Cucumbers are hydrating and contain antioxidants that help to reduce inflammation. Spinach is a great source of iron, calcium, and vitamins A and C. Green apples are rich in fiber and antioxidants. At the same time, lime provides additional vitamin C and adds a zesty flavor to the drink. Drinking this Emerald Elixir regularly can help to alkalize the body, boost the immune system, and promote healthy digestion.

- **Citrus Zinger: A mix of grapefruit, lemon, and ginger for a tart and tangy drink high in vitamin C and anti-inflammatory compounds.**

Citrus Zinger Recipe:

Ingredients:

- 2 grapefruits, peeled and segmented
- 1 lemon, peeled
- 1-inch piece of fresh ginger, peeled
- 1 cup of water
- Ice (optional)

Instructions:

1. Juice the grapefruits, lemon, and ginger in a juicer.
2. In a blender, combine the juice with water and blend until well combined.
3. Pour into glasses over ice, if desired.
4. Serve and enjoy!

This zesty and refreshing juice is not only a delicious way to start your day, but it's also packed with immune-boosting vitamin C and anti-inflammatory ginger, making it a great choice for cancer patients looking to support their overall health and well-being.

- **Garden Goddess: A combination of kale, cucumber, celery, green apple, and lemon for a nutrient-packed and alkalizing drink that supports overall health and well-being.**

Garden Goddess Juice Recipe:

Ingredients:

- 2 cups kale leaves
- 1 medium cucumber
- 3 stalks celery
- 1 green apple
- 1/2 lemon

Instructions:

1. Wash all the ingredients thoroughly.
2. Cut the cucumber, celery, and apple into small pieces.
3. Squeeze the juice out of the lemon.
4. Add all the ingredients to a juicer and process until smooth.
5. Pour the juice into a glass and enjoy immediately.

This nutrient-dense juice is packed with vitamins, minerals, and antioxidants that help to support overall health and well-being. The kale, cucumber, and celery are alkalizing and detoxifying, while the green apple adds a touch of sweetness and extra vitamins.

The lemon provides a burst of vitamin C and helps to balance the flavors of the other ingredients. Drink this Garden Goddess juice regularly to boost your immune system and promote optimal health.

- **Cherry Crush: A mix of cherries, pomegranate, and ginger for a delicious and antioxidant-rich drink that supports the immune system and helps to reduce inflammation.**

To make a Cherry Crush juice, you will need:

- 1 cup of pitted cherries
- 1/2 cup of pomegranate seeds
- 1-inch piece of ginger, peeled
- 1/2 cup of water

Instructions:

1. Wash and pit the cherries.
2. Cut the pomegranate in half and use a spoon to scoop out the seeds.
3. Peel the ginger and cut it into small pieces.
4. Add the cherries, pomegranate seeds, and ginger to a juicer.
5. Juice the ingredients according to the juicer's instructions.
6. Add water to the juice and mix well.
7. Pour the juice into a glass and enjoy!

Benefits:

Cherries are rich in antioxidants and have been shown to have anti-inflammatory properties. Pomegranate seeds are also high in antioxidants and may help to reduce inflammation in the body. Ginger is a natural anti-inflammatory and can help to soothe digestive issues. This juice is a delicious and nutrient-rich way to support the immune system and promote overall health and well-being.

- **Beet the Odds: A combination of beets, carrots, and apples for a high-nitrate drink that helps to lower blood pressure and supports overall cardiovascular health.**

Ingredients:

- 2 medium beets, peeled and chopped
- 3 medium carrots, peeled and chopped
- 2 medium apples, cored and chopped

Instructions:

1. Wash and prepare all the ingredients.
2. Juice the beets, carrots, and apples in a juicer.
3. Stir the juice well and serve immediately.

This drink is high in nitrates, converted to nitric oxide in the body. Nitric oxide helps to relax blood vessels, which helps lower blood pressure and improve overall cardiovascular health. Beets are also high in antioxidants and anti-inflammatory compounds, making this drink a great choice to boost your overall health and well-being.

- **Pineapple Ginger Zest: A mix of pineapple, ginger, and lime for a refreshing and energizing drink that supports digestion and reduces inflammation.**

To prepare the Pineapple Ginger Zest juice, you will need:

- 1 cup of fresh pineapple chunks
- 1-inch piece of fresh ginger root, peeled
- 1 lime, peeled
- 1/2 cup of water (or more, as needed)

Instructions:

1. Wash the pineapple and ginger root and peel the ginger.
2. Cut the pineapple into small chunks.
3. Cut the lime into quarters.
4. Add the pineapple, ginger, and lime to your juicer.
5. Turn on the juicer and extract the juice.
6. Add water as needed to thin the juice to your desired consistency.
7. Pour into a glass and serve immediately.

This juice is packed with antioxidants and anti-inflammatory compounds from the pineapple and ginger, while the lime provides a dose of vitamin C. The ginger also aids in digestion and can help to reduce inflammation in the body.

- **Blueberry Bliss: A blend of blueberries, strawberries, and raspberries for a delicious and high-antioxidant drink that supports the immune system and helps to fight against cancer.**

Ingredients:

- 1 cup blueberries
- 1 cup strawberries
- 1 cup raspberries
- 1/2 cup coconut water
- 1/2 cup plain Greek yogurt
- 1 tsp honey (optional)

Instructions:

1. Wash all the berries and remove any stems.

2. Add the berries, coconut water, Greek yogurt, and honey (if using) to a blender.
3. Blend until smooth and creamy.
4. Pour into a glass and enjoy immediately.

This delicious and nutritious juice is packed with antioxidants from the three types of berries, which help to support the immune system and fight against cancer. Adding coconut water and Greek yogurt provides hydration and protein, while the honey adds sweetness.

- **Topaz Tonic: A combination of green apple, cucumber, lemon, and ginger for a refreshing and detoxifying drink that supports liver function and overall well-being.**

Topaz Tonic Recipe:

Ingredients:

- 2 green apples, cored and sliced
- 1 medium cucumber, chopped
- 1 lemon, peeled and sliced
- 1-inch piece of ginger, peeled and sliced

Instructions:

1. Wash all the ingredients properly.
2. Cut the apples and cucumber into small pieces.
3. Peel the lemon and ginger and cut them into small pieces.
4. Add all the ingredients to the juicer.
5. Process until you have a smooth and consistent juice.
6. Serve immediately and enjoy.

Benefits:

This Topaz Tonic is a refreshing and detoxifying drink that can help to support liver function and overall well-being. The green apple provides a sweet and tart flavor, while the cucumber adds a refreshing and hydrating element. The lemon and ginger add a zesty and tangy kick while also providing detoxifying and anti-inflammatory benefits. This juice can be a great addition to a cancer patient's diet as it helps to support their body's natural detoxification process and overall health.

- **Aquamarine Elixir: A mix of pineapple, cucumber, and mint for a hydrating and anti-inflammatory drink that supports digestive health and overall wellness.**

Aquamarine Elixir Recipe:

Ingredients:

- 1 cup pineapple chunks
- 1 cucumber
- Handful of fresh mint leaves
- 1/2 cup water

Instructions:

1. Wash the pineapple, cucumber, and mint leaves thoroughly.
2. Cut the pineapple into chunks and peel the cucumber.
3. Add the pineapple, cucumber, and mint leaves into a juicer and juice them.
4. Pour the juice into a glass and stir in 1/2 cup of water.
5. Serve the Aquamarine Elixir chilled or over ice.

Benefits:

This refreshing and hydrating juice is packed with anti-inflammatory compounds that help to reduce inflammation and support overall wellness. Pineapple is rich in bromelain, an enzyme that aids digestion and reduces inflammation, while cucumber is a great source of hydration and contains anti-inflammatory flavonoids. Mint leaves provide a refreshing flavor and can also help to soothe the digestive system. Enjoy this Aquamarine Elixir as a part of a healthy diet to support digestive health and overall well-being.

- **Opal Oasis: A blend of watermelon, lime, and basil for a refreshing and hydrating drink that supports immune function and helps to reduce inflammation.**

Opal Oasis Recipe:

Ingredients:

- 4 cups of diced watermelon
- Juice of 1 lime
- 1/4 cup of fresh basil leaves

- 1/2 cup of ice

Instructions:

1. Add the watermelon, lime juice, and fresh basil to a blender.
2. Blend on high until the mixture is smooth.
3. Add the ice to the blender and blend again until the ice is crushed and the mixture is slushy.
4. Pour the Opal Oasis juice into glasses and serve immediately.

Opal Oasis is a refreshing and hydrating drink perfect for hot summer days. Watermelon is rich in antioxidants and contains high levels of vitamins A and C, which help to support immune function and protect against cancer.

Lime provides additional vitamin C and adds a tart and tangy flavor, while basil adds a fresh and herbaceous note to the drink. Enjoy this delicious and healthy juice as a snack or a post-workout drink to rehydrate and replenish your body.

- **Turquoise Temptation: A combination of kale, blueberries, and ginger for a high-antioxidant and anti-inflammatory drink that supports brain health and helps to fight against cancer.**

Turquoise Temptation Recipe:

Ingredients:

- 1 cup kale leaves
- 1 cup blueberries
- 1-inch ginger root
- 1/2 cup water

Instructions:

1. Wash and chop the kale leaves into small pieces.
2. Rinse the blueberries and set aside.
3. Peel the ginger root and cut it into small pieces.
4. Add all the ingredients into a juicer and blend until smooth.
5. If the mixture is too thick, add more water and blend again.
6. Pour the juice into a glass and serve immediately.

Turquoise Temptation is a delicious and nutritious juice that combines the health benefits of kale, blueberries, and ginger. Kale is rich in vitamins, minerals, and antioxidants that help support brain health and reduce cancer risk. Blueberries are also packed with antioxidants that help to boost the immune system and fight against cancer. Ginger is known for its anti-inflammatory properties and helps to soothe the digestive system. This juice is a perfect way to start your day and boost your health!

- **Emerald Empowerment: A mix of spinach, green apple, celery, and lemon for a nutrient-dense and alkalizing drink that supports overall health and well-being.**

Emerald Empowerment is a refreshing and nutrient-packed drink that will revitalize and empower you. This drink mixes spinach, green apple, celery, and lemon, providing many health benefits.

Spinach is rich in antioxidants and vitamins, including vitamin C and vitamin K. It also contains iron, which helps to support healthy blood cells and oxygen transport in the body. Green apples add a touch of sweetness and are high in fiber, which supports healthy digestion and helps to regulate blood sugar levels.

Celery is a low-calorie and hydrating vegetable rich in vitamins and minerals, including vitamin K, folate, and potassium. It also contains anti-inflammatory compounds that help to reduce inflammation in the body. Lemon adds a burst of tangy flavor and is high in vitamin C, which supports immune function and helps to protect against oxidative damage.

To make Emerald Empowerment, blend a handful of spinach, one green apple, two celery stalks, and the juice of one lemon. Add water as needed to achieve your desired consistency. This drink is perfect for any time of day and is a great way to start your morning or recharge after a workout.

Conclusion

In conclusion, the recipes presented here offer delicious and nutritious meals and specific benefits to you. The ingredients used in these recipes are rich in vitamins, minerals, and antioxidants that can help strengthen the immune system and reduce inflammation. Furthermore, these recipes are designed to be gentle on the stomach and easy to digest, making them an ideal choice for those experiencing nausea, vomiting, or other digestive issues.

By incorporating these recipes into your diet, you can provide vital nutritional support during treatment and recovery. Moreover, these recipes are versatile and can be adapted to meet your unique needs and preferences. So, take the first step towards improving your health by trying out these recipes.

Remember, your health is precious, and every small step you take towards better health counts towards your recovery. Juicing can offer you numerous benefits, such as increased energy, improved digestion, and radiant skin. Don't wait until it's too late to start taking care of your body. Begin juicing today and witness the transformation that awaits you. Invest in your health, and let the power of juicing work its healing power to transform your life.

- **Tips For Selecting The Best Produce And Storing It**

Selecting and storing the right produce correctly is essential for making healthy and delicious juices. Here are some tips for selecting the best produce and storing it:

1. **Choose fresh, ripe produce:** Choose items that are firm, ripe, and vibrant in color. Look for fruits and vegetables free from bruises, cuts, or any other signs of damage.

2. **Buy organic when possible:** Organic produce is free from harmful pesticides and chemicals that can harm your health. Whenever possible, choose organic produce for your juicing recipes.

3. **Seasonal produce:** Select produce in season for the best flavor and nutrition. It's also more affordable and widely available during peak seasons.

4. **Use a variety of produce:** Incorporate a variety of fruits and vegetables in your juices to maximize the nutrients you receive. Don't be afraid to mix and match different flavors and textures.

5. **Store produce correctly:** Store your produce in a cool, dry place, away from direct sunlight. Most fruits and vegetables

can be stored in the refrigerator in a crisper drawer to extend their shelf life.

6. **Wash produce thoroughly:** Before juicing, wash your produce thoroughly to remove any dirt or debris; this will help reduce the risk of foodborne illness.

7. **Use produce soon after purchase:** For the best flavor and nutrition, it's best to use your product soon after purchasing it. As fruits and vegetables age, their nutrient content decreases, and they may not taste as fresh.

Following these tips for selecting and storing produce can ensure your juices are delicious and nutritious.

- **Suggestions For Adjusting Recipes To Fit Your Need**

When it comes to juicing, there are many different recipes to choose from, but not every recipe will work for everyone. Here are some suggestions for adjusting recipes to fit your individual needs and preferences:

1. **Substitute fruits and vegetables:** If a recipe calls for an ingredient that you don't like or can't find, consider substituting it with something else. For

example, if a recipe calls for kale but you don't like the taste, you can substitute it with spinach or Swiss chard.

2. **Adjust sweetness:** If a recipe is too sweet for your taste, you can reduce the number of sweet ingredients, such as apples or carrots, and increase the number of vegetables. Similarly, if a recipe is not sweet enough, you can add a bit more fruit or a natural sweetener like honey or maple syrup.

3. **Add protein:** If you need more protein in your diet, you can add ingredients like nuts, seeds, or protein powder to your juices. These will also help make your juices more filling and satisfying.

4. **Adjust consistency:** If you prefer your juices to be thicker or thinner, you can adjust the consistency by adding more or less water, or by using a different type of produce.

5. **Experiment with herbs and spices:** Adding herbs and spices like ginger, turmeric, or mint to your juices can add flavor and nutrition. Experiment with different combinations to find your favorites.

6. **Consider dietary restrictions:** If you have any dietary restrictions or food allergies, make sure to adjust recipes accordingly. For example, if you're lactose intolerant, you may need to avoid using dairy-based ingredients in your juices.

7. **Consult with a healthcare professional:** If you have specific health concerns or medical conditions, it's always a good idea to consult with a healthcare professional before making any dietary changes, including adding juicing to your diet.

By adjusting recipes to fit your individual needs and preferences, you can create delicious and nutritious juices that work for you. Don't be afraid to experiment and try new things until you find the perfect recipe for your taste buds and health goals.

Chapter 6

Integrating Juicing into Your Treatment Plan

IIntegrating juicing into your cancer treatment plan can benefit your health and well-being. This section will discuss guidelines for incorporating juicing into your treatment plan and offer tips for juicing while undergoing cancer treatment.

- **Guidelines For Incorporating Juicing Into Your Cancer Treatment Plan**

When incorporating juicing into your cancer treatment plan, it is essential to follow specific guidelines to ensure that you maximise the benefits and minimise any potential risks. Here are some general guidelines to keep in mind:

1. **Please consult with your doctor:** Before making any changes to your treatment plan, it is essential to consult with your doctor or a registered dietitian. They can advise you on whether juicing is safe and appropriate for your individual needs and offer suggestions for specific fruits and vegetables to include in your juices.

2. **Choose the right produce:** The right product is crucial for creating nutritious

and safe juices. Opt for organic produce when possible, and avoid any fruits or vegetables that may interact with your medications. Some medications can interact with certain fruits and vegetables, so you must talk to your doctor or a registered dietitian about potential interactions.

3. **Clean your produce thoroughly:** To reduce the risk of foodborne illness, thoroughly wash all produce before juicing; this can be done using a fruit and vegetable wash or simply rinsing them with cold water.

4. **Start slow:** If you are new to juicing or have a compromised immune system, it is essential to start slow and gradually increase the amount of juice you consume. Begin with a small amount, such as 4-6 ounces per day, and slowly increase over time.

5. **Monitor your blood sugar:** Some juices can be high in sugar, which can cause spikes in blood sugar levels. Suppose you have diabetes or are at risk of developing it. In that case, it is essential to monitor your blood sugar levels and choose juices that are lower in sugar or contain

ingredients that can help regulate blood sugar.

6. **Be mindful of calories:** Juicing can be a great way to increase your intake of nutrients, but it is essential to be mindful of the number of calories you consume. Juices high in fruits can be exceptionally high in calories, so try to balance them with lower-calorie vegetables or use smaller amounts of fruit.

By following these guidelines, you can incorporate juicing into your cancer treatment plan safely and effectively. Before changing your treatment plan, remember to consult your doctor or a registered dietitian. Listen to your body to determine what works best for you.

- **Tips For Juicing While Undergoing Cancer Treatment, Including Addressing Common Concerns Such As Taste Changes And Digestion Issues**

Juicing is an effective way to supplement cancer treatment, providing the body with vital nutrients that support the immune system and help fight cancer. However, undergoing cancer treatment can come with a range of challenges, including changes in taste preferences and digestive issues.

Here are some tips for juicing while undergoing cancer treatment:

1. **Start slow:** If you are new to juicing, start with small amounts and gradually increase the amount of juice you consume. This will help your body adjust to the influx of nutrients.

2. **Experiment with different recipes:** Taste changes are common during cancer treatment, and some juices may taste better than others. Experiment with different recipes and find the ones that you enjoy the most.

3. **Use fresh, organic produce:** Opt for fresh, organic produce whenever possible, as it is free from harmful pesticides and chemicals.

4. **Consider digestive enzymes:** If you experience digestive issues while juicing, consider adding digestive enzymes to your diet to help your body break down the nutrients.

5. **Talk to your doctor:** If you are concerned about how juicing may interact with your treatment plan or medications, speak with your doctor or a registered dietitian.

6. **Use a slow juicer:** A slow juicer extracts more nutrients and enzymes from fruits and vegetables, making the juice more nutrient-dense and easier to digest.

7. **Hydrate:** Drinking plenty of water is important when juicing, as it helps flush toxins out of the body and prevents dehydration.

8. **Consider the time of day:** Drinking juice on an empty stomach can be more beneficial for absorption, but if you experience nausea or digestive issues, you may want to try drinking juice with a small meal or snack.

In summary, juicing can be a valuable addition to a cancer treatment plan, but it's important to take into account any taste changes and digestive issues that may arise. By starting slow, experimenting with different recipes, and staying hydrated, you can incorporate juicing into your cancer treatment plan and reap the benefits of its nutrient-rich goodness.

Chapter 7

Conclusion

In conclusion, incorporating juicing into a cancer treatment plan will benefit you. Juicing is a powerful complementary therapy, from boosting the immune system and fighting inflammation to detoxifying the body and providing essential nutrients.

You can safely and effectively incorporate juicing into your treatment plan by selecting the best produce, adjusting recipes to fit individual needs, and addressing concerns such as taste changes and digestion issues.

- **Recap of the benefits of juicing in cancer treatment**

In conclusion, juicing is a valuable complementary treatment for you. By providing essential nutrients, antioxidants, and anti-inflammatory compounds, juicing will help boost your immune system, reduce inflammation, and fight cancer cells.

Green, immune-boosting, antioxidant-rich, and detoxifying juices can provide specific benefits for cancer patients. Additionally, you can safely and effectively incorporate juicing into your treatment plan by following guidelines for selecting and storing produce, adjusting recipes to fit your need, and addressing common concerns like taste changes and digestion issues.

So if you or a loved one are undergoing cancer treatment, consider incorporating juicing to support overall health and well-being.

- **Final Thoughts And Encouragement For You To Try Juicing**

In conclusion, incorporating juicing into a cancer treatment plan will benefit you. Juicing offers a convenient and effective way to consume essential nutrients that will help boost your immune system, fight inflammation, detoxify the body, and promote overall health and well-being.

While juicing is not a cure for cancer, it will serve as a valuable complementary therapy to traditional treatments. It is essential to consult with a healthcare professional before starting a juicing regimen, especially if you are undergoing cancer treatment or taking medications.

As we conclude, the benefits of incorporating juicing into the diet of cancer patients cannot be overstated. The recipes presented here are delicious and packed with the vital nutrients, vitamins, and antioxidants your body needs to strengthen the immune system and reduce inflammation.

We understand that cancer can be challenging, and with the recipes in this book, it will be a lot easier.

Remember, you are not alone in this fight; every small step you take toward better health counts. Try juicing and see its transformative impact on your physical and mental well-being. Stay positive, stay motivated, and keep fighting, for the **power to heal and overcome cancer lies within you.**

- **Additional Resources For Juicing And Cancer Support**

If you're interested in learning more about juicing and cancer support, there are several resources available:

1. **American Institute for Cancer Research (AICR):** AICR offers a variety of resources on nutrition and cancer prevention, including information on juicing and cancer.
2. **American Cancer Society (ACS):** The ACS provides resources for cancer patients and their families, including information on nutrition during cancer treatment.
3. **Juicing for Health:** This website offers a variety of juicing recipes and information on the health benefits of juicing.
4. **National Cancer Institute (NCI):** The NCI offers information on cancer treatment and support, as well as nutrition and dietary guidance for cancer patients.
5. **Cancer Support Community:** The Cancer Support Community provides resources and support for cancer patients and their families, including information on nutrition and lifestyle choices.
6. **Integrative Oncology Essentials:** This website provides information on integrative approaches to cancer treatment, including nutrition and lifestyle choices.

Incorporating juicing into your cancer treatment plan boosts your immune system, fights inflammation, and reduces the risk of cancer recurrence. **Remember to prioritize a balanced diet, physical activity, and other lifestyle factors to support your overall health and well-being.**

Cheers to a healthier you!

Detox, nourish yourself.

Beat Cancer with Anti-Cancer Juicing Recipes: 150+ Mouthwatering Recipes for Detox and Nourishment!

www.ingramcontent.com/pod-product-compliance
Lightning Source LLC
Chambersburg PA
CBHW061624250726

48659CB00004B/1077